CLINICAL METHODS IN DENTAL OFFICE

History Recording, Examination, Investigations and Therapeutics

CLINICAL METHODS IN DENTAL OFFICE

History Recording, Examination, Investigations and Therapeutics

Santosh Patil BDS MDS
Reader
Department of Oral Medicine and Radiology
Jodhpur Dental College General Hospital
Jodhpur, Rajasthan, India

Sneha Maheshwari BDS FAGE
Dental Practitioner
Jodhpur, Rajasthan, India

Foreword

Bader K Alzarea

JAYPEE *The Health Sciences Publisher*
New Delhi | London | Philadelphia | Panama

JAYPEE **Jaypee Brothers Medical Publishers (P) Ltd.**

Headquarters

Jaypee Brothers Medical Publishers (P) Ltd.
4838/24, Ansari Road, Daryaganj
New Delhi 110 002, India
Phone: +91-11-43574357
Fax: +91-11-43574314
E-mail: jaypee@jaypeebrothers.com

Overseas Offices

J.P. Medical Ltd.
83, Victoria Street, London
SW1H 0HW (UK)
Phone: +44-20 3170 8910
Fax: +44(0) 20 3008 6180
E-mail: info@jpmedpub.com

Jaypee-Highlights Medical Publishers Inc.
City of Knowledge
Building 235, 2nd Floor
Clayton, Panama City, Panama
Phone: +1 507-301-0496
Fax: +1 507-301-0499
E-mail: cservice@jphmedical.com

Jaypee Medical Inc.
325, Chestnut Street
Suite 412, Philadelphia
PA 19106 USA
Phone: +1 267-519-9789
E-mail: support@jpmedus.com

Jaypee Brothers Medical Publishers (P) Ltd.
17/1-B, Babar Road, Block-B
Shaymali, Mohammadpur
Dhaka-1207, Bangladesh
Mobile: +08801912003485
E-mail: jaypeedhaka@gmail.com

Jaypee Brothers Medical Publishers (P) Ltd.
Bhotahity, Kathmandu, Nepal
Phone: +977-9741283608
E-mail: kathmandu@jaypeebrothers.com

Website: www.jaypeebrothers.com
Website: www.jaypeedigital.com

Inquiries for bulk sales may be solicited at: jaypee@jaypeebrothers.com

Clinical Methods in Dental Office: History Recording, Examination, Investigations and Therapeutics

First Edition : **2017**

ISBN 978-93-86150-02-8

Printed at Sanat Printers

Dedicated to

The people who showed us this world and to those who stood by in the journey.

Kingdom of Saudi Arabia Ministry of Education
Aljouf University
College of Dentistry

بسم الله الرحمن الرحيم

المملكة العربية السعودية
وزارة التعليم
جامعة الجوف
كلية طب الأسنان

Foreword

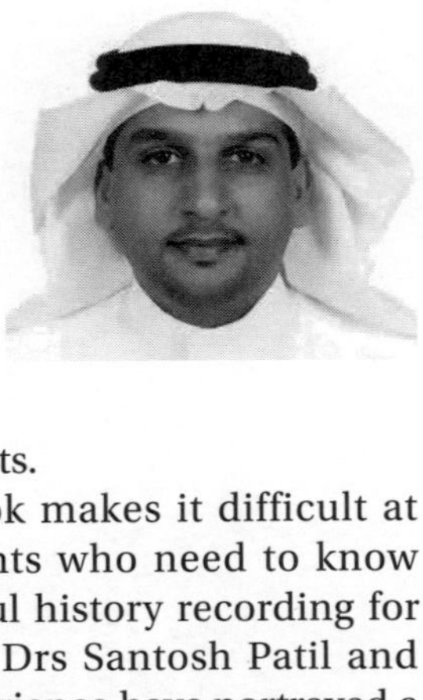

Clinical Methods in Dental Office: History Recording, Examination, Investigations and Therapeutics seeks to assist dental students, dentists and dental assistants to make informed clinical decisions on the optimal examination, diagnosis and treatment plan of the patients. As active academic clinicians, we continue to seek educational formats that reconcile clinical research development with a provocative pedagogical approach on which never loses sight of those who benefit most from our service—our patients.

The lack of a comprehensive and precise book makes it difficult at undergraduate level, especially for dental students who need to know basic examination principles in general and careful history recording for accurate diagnosis and management of patients. Drs Santosh Patil and Sneha Maheshwari with tremendous effort and experience have portrayed a manual, which will be of immense help to the dental students, postgraduates and clinicians in their clinical examinations and understanding the patients' problems in a simple manner.

I am sure that their contribution to the profession will be greatly appreciated by all professional colleagues. I wish them success in their noble but humble mission.

Bader K Alzarea
Dean
College of Dentistry
Al Jouf University
Al-Jawf
Kingdom of Saudia Arabia

Preface

Clinical Methods in Dental Office: History Recording, Examination, Investigations and Therapeutics is intended to provide insight into the realms of the clinical aspects of oral medicine and radiology to the student entering dental clinics for the first time. The undergraduates begin with their clinical training in the third year of the BDS curriculum, where they interact and evaluate patients for the very first time. The book will help the students in understanding the patient's orofacial complaints and the subsequent step-by-step examination of oral and paraoral structures. It will also serve as a ready-reckoner for private dental practitioners and postgraduate dental students.

The book describes history taking for regular and special cases. It also prepares and sensitizes the students to the needs of patients with certain mental and physical disabilities, individuals with underlying systemic diseases and handling of medical emergencies in the dental clinics and offices. It also contains the commonly used medications for various oral conditions, which will help students and practitioners to use it as a ready reference while prescribing drugs to the patients. Also, a chapter on the various laboratory and radiographic investigations will help the students and practitioners in formulating an accurate diagnosis by the selection of the most appropriate investigations.

It is our hope that the presentation of the fundamental basis of case history recordings, examinations, investigations and therapeutics will be useful to the students and practitioners and that it will contribute to the continuous progress of the profession.

Santosh Patil
Sneha Maheshwari

Acknowledgments

Writing *Clinical Methods in Dental Office: History Recording, Examination, Investigations and Therapeutics* happens to be one of the greatest achievements in our lives. We readily acknowledge our indebtedness to the many teachers, colleagues and friends with whose influence over the years, sincere and enthusiastic support, we have been able to write this book. They together with our technicians, assistants and patients, are the ones who really made this text possible. The immense knowledge and experience of all these individuals adds immeasurably to the text.

We are also grateful for the skillful and generous support from the staff at M/s Jaypee Brothers Medical Publishers (P) Ltd, New Delhi, India, for their energy and creativity in the presentation of the content.

Contents

1. Oral Medicine and Oral Diagnosis: Introduction and Scope 1

2. History and Definitions 3

- Definitions 3

3. Significance of Patient's History Recording 5

- Definition 5
- Types of Case History 6
- Principles of Examination of Patient 7
- Starting the Consultation 8
- Personal Identification Data 10
- Chief Complaint 12
- History of Present Illness 13
- Past Dental History 14
- Past Medical History 14
- Cardiovascular System 15
- Respiratory System 17
- Gastrointestinal System 17
- Endocrine System 18
- Hematopoietic 18
- Musculoskeletal System 19
- Neurologic System 19
- Cranial Nerve Examination 20
- Genitourinary 22
- Blood Transfusions 22
- Allergies 22
- Pregnancy 23
- Medications 23
- Family History 23
- Personal History 24
- Habits Related to Oral Cavity 25
- Dietary Habit 26

4. General Physical Examination of Patient 27

- General Examination 28
- Vital Signs 29
- Signs of Anemia 32
- Signs of Cyanosis 33
- Eyes 33
- Nose 34
- Extremities 35
- Nails 35
- Skin 36

5. **Examination of Head and Neck Region** **38**
- Facial Appearance in Different Diseases 39
- Temporomandibular Joint Examination 39
- Muscles of Mastication 41
- Examination of the Neck 42
- Intraoral Examination 46
- Anomalies of the Tongue 49
- Hard Tissue Examination 55
- Tooth Wear 59
- Discoloration of Teeth 59
- Dental Caries 60
- Occlusion 61
- Examination of Swelling 62
- Examination of an Ulcer 63

6. **Investigations** **67**
- Plaque Disclosing Agents 69
- Caries Detecting Dyes 69
- Pulp Vitality Tests 70
- Uses of Pulp Vitality Testing 70
- Toludine Blue and Lugol's Iodine Staining 75
- Salivary Flow Test 76
- Diagnostic Nerve Blocking 77
- Antibiotic Sensitivity Test 77
- Diascopic Examination 78
- Hematological Investigations 78
- Estimation of Blood Sugar 88
- Glycosylated Hemoglobin 91
- Microbiological Investigations 92
- Isolation of the Oral Microbial Flora 93
- Specimen Collection and Procedure 93
- Cultures of Tooth Apices 94
- Bacterial Cultures in Endodontics 94
- Examination of Microbial Flora from Plaque and Gingival Crevice 95
- Caries Activity Tests 95
- Biopsy 98
- Fine Needle Aspiration Biopsy 99
- Exfoliative Cytology 101
- Punch Biopsy 102
- Brush Biopsy 103
- Types of Artifacts 104
- Frozen Sections 105
- Sialochemical Investigations 106
- Serology 108
- Cytogenetics and Chromosome Analysis 111
- Maxillofacial Imaging 111
- Temporomandibular Joint Radiography 115
- Hard Tissue Imaging 116
- Soft Tissue Imaging 117
- Ultrasonography 117

• Nuclear Medicine 118
• Imaging for Salivary Gland Diseases 118

7. Therapeutics **120**

• Treatment of Common Oral Diseases 128
• Complementary and Alternative Medicine Techniques Available for Dentistry 138

8. Guidelines for Management of Medically Compromised Patients in Dental Office **146**

• Diabetes Mellitus 147
• Anemia 150
• Epilepsy 152
• Bronchial Asthma 152
• Renal Diseases 153
• Liver Disorders 153
• Hepatitis B 154
• Patients Receiving Steroid Therapy 155
• General Guidelines 155
• HIV and AIDS 160
• Tuberculosis 160

9. Management of Medical Emergencies **161**

• Patient History 162
• Office Emergency Plan 162
• Emergency Training 164
• Initial Emergency Procedures 165
• Anxiety Reduction 167
• Anaphylaxis 168
• Mild Allergy 168
• Asthma 169
• Angina and Myocardial Infarction 170
• Cardiac Arrest 171
• Epilepsy 171
• Syncope 172
• Hypoglycemia 173
• Accidental Overdose 174

10. Checklist for Recording Patient's Data **175**

Annexure *185*

Glossary *203*

Bibliography *231*

Index *243*

1

Oral Medicine and Oral Diagnosis: Introduction and Scope

Sir Jonathan Hutchinson (1828–1900), surgeon to the London Hospital, regarded as Father of Oral Medicine said "Ever since man has been interested in his own health and health of his neighbors, he observed that appearance of skin may denote ill health with the cause sometimes readily ascertained by examining the oral cavity and in particular tongue and gums. Thus all physicians have and still do practice oral medicine."

Prevalence of medical disorders influencing dental treatment has relatively increased in the modern times. The branch of oral medicine is considered as an interface between general medicine and dentistry. It has now become necessary to identify the presence and significance of medical problems that are likely to affect the dental treatment, thus emphasizing the need for a good preoperative assessment.

As modern rational therapy is based upon the scientific interpretation of the changes in function and structure of the tissues of the body, the importance of an accurate diagnosis is hence evident. The basic principle of diagnosis is to observe and describe the alterations from the normal features, which is based on favorable interview and examination of the patient. There can be only one accurate diagnosis upon which the success of treatment is dependent. Therefore, in our endeavor to render the best possible service to the patient every known method should be employed, if necessary, in making an accurate diagnosis. It must be emphasized that examination of supposedly healthy mouth must be thorough and careful, since the early detection of disease demands that slightest of the details of any deviations be carefully evaluated.

No one other than a qualified dentist, well-trained in the field of oral medicine has the ability to diagnose oral lesions, to consult and interact with appropriate medical practitioners for planning and carrying out dental treatment for medically compromised patients. Method of systematic observation and description is the foundation of oral diagnosis. The ability to take an accurate history from a patient is one of the core clinical skills and an essential component of clinical competence. The interview or consultation influences the precision of diagnosis and treatment, and various studies have indicated that over 80% of diagnoses in general dental clinics are based on the accurate history recording. With this basic knowledge and concept in mind; dental practitioners should broaden their interest in formulating a true diagnosis and the formulation of a corresponding treatment plan and thus, encourage the patients towards the maintenance of a good oral health.

The field is extensive and its scope is not unlike other specialized fields in dentistry. It comprises of the diagnosis and treatment of oral mucosal diseases, other oral complains that may reflect either local oral diseases or oral manifestations of systemic diseases and phases of dental practice especially concerned with physiologically compromised patients. The practice of oral diagnosis/oral medicine includes the application of the knowledge of pathophysiology of disease, pharmacotherapeutics, and dental sciences that leads to formulation of a diagnosis, management of the disease and patient health maintenance. An unusual amount of training and specialized skill are required to diagnose and treat oral diseases, and for this reason it is not practical for the general practitioners of medicine or dentistry to have a very comprehensive knowledge of oral disease. Hence, the role of physicians specialized in the field of oral medicine includes:

- The role as a consultant to private practitioners for diagnostic and treatment planning.
- They should be able to provide a variety of therapeutic measures for the patients with common and rare oral health problems.
- They should serve as a mediator between fellow dentists and their medical counter parts, particularly in the fields of otorhinolaryngology, dermatology, neurology, pharmacology, internal medicine, oncology and radiology.
- They should be able to design and execute clinical research directed towards increasing present knowledge or introducing new therapeutic modalities for oral diseases.
- They should demonstrate increased knowledge and competency in oral diagnosis/oral medicine, particularly in the application and promotion of newer diagnostic techniques and therapeutic measures.

The importance of oral diagnosis in preventive dentistry can be appreciated by the fact that the prevention of diseases is based upon thorough examination of all the patients, which can be achieved through correct diagnosis of patients' oral disease. Even in making an examination for the diagnosis of a local condition the field of observation must be broad. The examiner should be alert to general conditions that indirectly influence the oral lesion. Hence, diagnosis requires a broad general concept of oral diseases and an appreciation of the relationship of oral diseases to other disorders of the body.

2

History and Definitions

The field of oral medicine took long to be recognized as a specialist discipline in dentistry. During 19th century only dermatology books described oral mucosal diseases in detail. It was through the efforts of Sir Jonathan Hutchinson (1828–1900) that a number of conditions of great interest to those working in the field of oral medicine, such as dental manifestation of syphilis acquired in utero; and intraoral pigmentation associated with circumoral pigmentation were discussed in detail. Later these were described by Peutz and Jegher. Henry T Butlin, in 1885 wrote a book titled 'Diseases of the Tongue'.

William Hunter through his publication in 1911, accused conservative dentistry and prosthetics for being the cause of oral sepsis, which in turn resulted in rheumatic and other chronic disease. Kenneth Goadby, in 1923 wrote his book entitled 'Diseases of the Gums and Oral Mucous Membrane'. FW Broderick published his book entitled 'Dental Medicine' in 1928 and attempted to introduce the biochemical basis for an understanding of dental disease. Kurt Thoma, published two book entitled 'Diagnosis and Treatment Planning' in 1938 and 'Oral Pathology' in 1941.

Lester Burkett, is famously known for publishing the first book completely dedicated to oral medicine in 1946. Hubert Stones, in 1948 published his book entitled 'Oral and Dental Diseases'. HM Worth, in 1963 wrote his book entitled 'The Principles and Practice of Oral Radiologic Interpretation'. The Nuffield foundation financed the chair in oral medicine at Newcastle for 10 years and John Boyes, in 1958 shifted the chair to dental surgery in Edinburgh. Later on Martin Rushton attracted young research workers and others interested in the field of oral medicine and oral pathology, and his influence is felt in many oral medicine departments today.

Definitions

Diagnosis is defined as the art and science of recognizing the presence and nature of disease by an evaluation of its various distinctive signs, symptoms and characteristics. It is a Greek word derived from 2 words 'dia' and 'gnosis' meaning through knowledge. Various definitions have been proposed by different authors as under:

- According to Zegarelli Edward V (1972), diagnosis is defined as the ability of the clinician to recognize and identify a specific abnormality and the ability to give a name to the disease process.

- Halstead Charles L (1982) defined diagnosis as the process of determining the nature of abnormality or disease that is producing signs/symptoms or both.
- Kerr Ash Millard (6th edition) defined diagnosis as the identification of oral diseases by interviewing, examining and synthesizing the descriptive features of the diseases and facts obtained from examination and interview.

Oral medicine is a specialized area of study within the scope of dental medicine. It is the interface between dentistry and medicine. The field of oral medicine consists primarily of the diagnosis and medical management of the patient with complex medical disorders involving the oral mucosa and salivary glands as well as orofacial pain and temporomandibular disorders.

The American Academy of Oral Medicine defines the field as follows:

- Oral medicine is the speciality of dentistry that is concerned with the oral health care of medically compromised patients and with the diagnosis and nonsurgical management of medically related disorders or conditions affecting the oral and maxillofacial region.
- According to Chrisholm Derric H et al. (1978) oral medicine is that part of dentistry that is involved in diagnosis and treatment of oral diseases of nonsurgical nature which may be localized to mouth or which may be oral manifestations of systemic diseases.
- Eversole in 1984 defined oral medicine as the discipline that subsumes internal medicine as it impacts on dental care management of medically ill patients, diagnosis of systemic diseases on the basis of oral head and neck manifestations, diagnosis and management of oral soft tissue diseases and diagnosis and management of facial pain.
- Williams R Tyldesley (1989) defined oral medicine as concerned with study and nonsurgical treatment of diseases affecting oral cavity and related structures.
- The triple O in 1992 defined oral medicine as that area of special competence in dentistry concerned with diseases that involve oral and paraoral structures especially oral manifestations of systemic diseases and behavioral disorders and oral and dental treatment of medically compromised patients.
- According to Burket's (11th edition) oral medicine is a clinical discipline with in dentistry that encompasses the following:
  - Diagnosis and medical management of diseases of oral mucosa, jaws and salivary glands.
  - Diagnosis and medical management of facial pain and temporomandibular joint diseases.
  - Dental treatment of patients with complicating medical diseases.

3

Significance of Patient's History Recording

You are likely to have heard this during your first clinical postings 'There is no such thing as a poor historian, just a poor history taker.' This is true to a great extent. We have to learn the topics we need information on and the different ways of obtaining that information. Good clinical assessment is the cornerstone of good practice and underpins the advanced practitioner's differential diagnosis and subsequent treatment plan and is one of the most rewarding aspects of patient care. It is the hallmark of a good clinician and is a skill which never dates.

Case history constitutes foundation not only for an intelligent approach to diagnosis but also for a successful patient-clinician relationship. It is based on the interview with the patient, where they should be encouraged to tell their story voluntarily. The clinician should only interrupt to obtain clarification of, or further information regarding specific points. The quality of history is largely determined by the competence of the interviewer but is also affected by the ability of the patient to communicate.

Definition

Case history is a planned professional conversation between patient and dentist which enables the patient to express his symptoms, fear and feelings to the clinician so that the nature of patient's real or suspected illness and mental attitude may be determined (Malcolm A Lynch).

Objectives of recording a case history:

- To formulate a pattern of asking relevant questions to get to the point data for the diagnosis as well as to alleviate the fear in the patient towards the disease and its treatment.
- To help in recording the intraoral and extraoral examination done based on the complaint of the patient.
- To record the specific intraoral lesions and extraoral lesions for the record purpose, diagnosis and effective treatment planning.
- Understanding the need for referral to other departments and the expectations of the outcome of the referral.

Objectives of case history will guide and improve the efforts of any examiner to:

- Arrive at a tentative diagnosis.
- Determine any systemic factors that might affect formulation of diagnosis.
- Determine any systemic conditions that require special precautions prior, to or during dental procedures to protect health and life of patient.

In addition, to the above benefits other advantages to the dentist include establishment of written records that will serve as a diagnostic instrument, protection from possible disease contact, establishment of a basis of future reference and provision of a document that will serve as a legal evidence for forensic odontology.

Types of Case History

1. *Structural case history:* Questions are asked in a logical manner according to a pre-decided format.
2. *Nonstructural case history:* Pattern of questions is changed according to patient's narration and there is no pre-decided format.

   The importance of case history taking in the practice of dental offices and clinics cannot be overestimated. In many instances the history of a case is relatively more important in making a diagnosis. In many cases a carefully taken history, including salient data, carefully written, and properly appraised will alone establish the diagnosis. This is notably true of tic douloureux in which the physical and laboratory findings are of little help and the diagnosis is made chiefly from the history. Hemophilia, hemorrhagic tendencies, cardiac disorders, lung disease, stomatitis due to drug poisoning and idiosyncrasies, heavy metal poisoning, salivary gland obstructions, vitamin deficiencies, neuralgias, early acute osteomyelitis, and early deep infections are only a few of the many conditions in which the history is an important factor in diagnosis.

Case history taking is an art, and science which takes into account the ingenuity, judgment and tact of clinical experience of the examiner to the fullest extent. The ones with extensive clinical experience record the most valuable case histories, as this enables them to search out and evaluate the most important facts in the case. A wide clinical experience is a necessary pre-requisite, of keen diagnostic ability, which is not always related to years of experience. One man, making full utilization of the senses of sight, touch, hearing and smell, can gain more experience in a year than another in a lifetime who looks but does not see, touches but does not feel, listens but does not hear, and smells but does not detect. A history may be valueless and extremely misleading if hurriedly taken and improperly recorded. The length of a history is by no means an indication of its value. It is better to have a short accurate concise statement containing the important facts regarding the case than a voluminous amount of extraneous material. A brief history containing salient facts is at once obviously more valuable than one written at length, but because of the inexperience of the questioner contains an abundance of irrelevant data presented in an incoherent manner. By brief proper queries, valuable information can be obtained without much loss of time. A proper knowledge of various diseases and conditions is necessary in order to determine the questions to be directed and in order to distinguish the relevant information from the irrelevant.

This may sound rather discouraging to the newcomers and inexperienced in the field. However, if a practice of taking routine histories in a careful, orderly, systematic manner is developed, it will be soon observed that it is not as difficult as it first appears. Careful case history taking aids in concluding a definite diagnosis, but also affords an adequate record system, the careful study of which will eventually result in the crystallizing of very definite ideas regarding the diagnosis and treatment plan of oral diseases.

Principles of Examination of Patient

Sir William Osler has said 'If you listen carefully to the patient they will tell you the diagnosis.'

How may you gain information from a patient? Visual and physical signs, obtained by examination of a patient, can be useful but the majority of information about a patient is obtained through verbal communication. Relevant and useful information can be obtained by careful and appropriate questioning. The type, quality and reliability of information gained by questioning a patient, friend or relative are dependent on how you ask the question in the first place. There are three major types of questions used in history-taking:

1. *Closed question:* A question that only gives a limited choice of answer, such as yes or no. For example: Do you have pain?
2. *Open question:* A question that can be answered freely, with as much or as little information as the responder wants to give. For example: What is troubling you at the moment?
3. *Probing questions:* These are more direct questions than open questions, as they are based on information already obtained but allow a free response. For example: In what way does your tooth pain affect your eating?

Where possible, ask open questions, especially at the start of the history. This makes it easier for patients to give accurate answers. Leading questions, like 'You do not have pain do you?' should not be asked. Such questions may lead to incorrect answers by the patients, because they may think it is what you want to hear. The timing of your questions is important. Multiple questions in one breath confuse patients and result in missed answers. You will feel like you are saving time but your history will not be as thorough. During the interview it is usual to use a combination of open-ended and closed questions. Normally, open questions are more commonly asked at the start of the interview with closed questions asked later, as information gathering becomes more focused in an attempt to elicit more detail.

Starting the Consultation

There are three main aspects to initiating the session: preparation, establishing initial rapport, and identifying the patient's problems and concerns.

Preparation

In preparing for a consultation, you should plan for an optimal setting to conduct the interview. In general practice or in the outpatient department, the consulting room should be quiet and free from interruptions. Patients often find that the clinical setting stokes up anxiety and therefore the environment should be made welcoming and relaxing. Time should be appropriately managed when preparing for the consultation. Ideally the practitioner should not appear rushed, and ensure that you set aside adequate time for the patient. The patient's first judgment is also influenced by the dress of the clinician. Fashions may change, but most patients have clear expectations of an appropriate dress and hence, it is advisable to adopt a dress code that projects a professional image. This may vary according to setting and patient group, like children may feel more comfortable with a doctor who adopts a slightly more informal appearance. Along with the attire, attention should be paid to personal hygiene; for example ensure that the hands and nails are clean.

Establishing an Initial Rapport

Creating a rapport with the patient and gaining their trust is a key skill when taking a history. This is not always possible due to the nature of the illness/ injury, communication difficulties or previous bad experience. It is a chance for you to demonstrate from the outset your respect, interest and concern for them. Before you start with the history taking, patient's consent should be gained. On approach, introduce yourself and explain that you are there to take care of them. It may sometimes be appropriate to give an idea of how long the interview might take. Patient-clinician communication consists not only of verbal discourse but also includes body language, especially facial expression and eye contact. When possible be at eye level while recording the history. The first contact should also be used to obtain or confirm the patient's name and to check how they prefer to be called. Some people are at ease when addressed by their first name, whilst others may prefer the use of their surname. If anybody is with the patient, ask who they are to the patient and if the patient is happy for them to stay in the room. State the need for the patient's history and what will be done with the information gained. Only then do you ask if it is ok to continue with the history.

Identifying the Problems and Concerns of the Patient

One of the most important factors in this relationship is letting the patient know that they have been heard, that you believe them and that you want what is best for them. Start by asking an open question relating to the presenting illness (e.g. What has brought you to the doctor today?). Allow for silences and use gentle encouragement to let them continue their story. Encourage the patient to describe how they feel, rather than tell you what someone else says is wrong with them. While open questions are always encouraged, there are times when closed questions are useful in the history or when the patient presents with multiple complaints (e.g. What is bothering you most at the moment?). The order of their problems may not relate to their importance from either the patient's or doctor's perspective. It is therefore particularly important in this initial phase not to interrupt the patient as this might inhibit the disclosure of important information. Try to avoid asking leading questions (e.g. Instead of asking Did the pain radiate into your neck and arm? You may ask Did the pain move?). Once the problems have been identified, it is worth reflecting on whether you have understood the patient correctly; which can be achieved by repeating the history to the patient. Closing the assessment with "Is there anything else you'd like to tell me?" is a good practice. A collateral history from relatives or friends, the patient's environment or apparent inconsistencies can inform the history. You may write down a summary of the patient's comments, but constantly maintain eye contact and avoid becoming too immersed in writing (or using a computer keyboard).

Gathering information on the patient's problems is one of the most important tasks to be mastered in clinical practice. The doctor must use a range of skills to encourage the patient to tell their complete information whilst maintaining a degree of control and a structure in the collection of information. As the history emerges, the doctor must interpret the symptom complex. The manner in which the interview is conducted, the conduct of the doctor and the type of questions asked may provide an insight on the information revealed by the patient. Obtaining all the relevant information from the patient can be decisive in formulating an accurate diagnosis **(Flow chart 1)**. The patient should feel that their welfare is central to the doctor's concern, that their complaint will be listened attentively, and their information and views will be highly valued. Since, most patients have no knowledge of anatomy, physiology or pathology, it is very important to use simple and patient friendly language and avoid medical terminologies.

Flow chart 1: Contents of case history

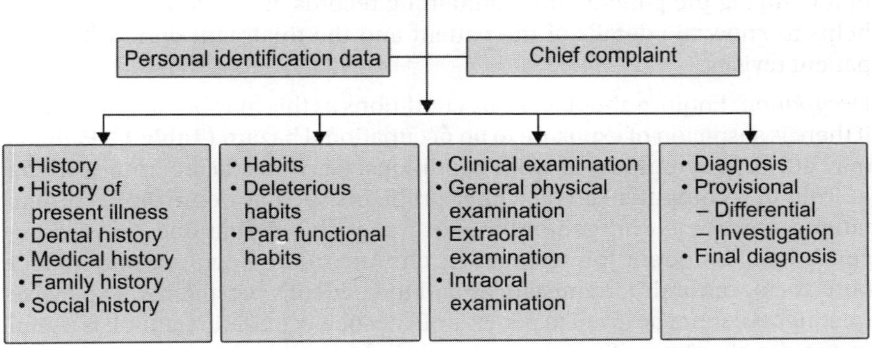

Personal Identification Data

Name: A patient usually likes to be called. It helps to elicit a better history and is of psychological benefit to the patients. This also helps in identification, record maintenance and communication when needed. Pediatric patients talk freely when addressed by their names or nicknames.

Age: Knowing the patient's age is important to the clinician as certain diseases are present at certain ages. For example

- Complete absence of teeth even at the age of 4–5 years is frequently associated with hereditary ectodermal dysplasia.
- Delayed eruption of teeth may be associated with rickets, cretinism or local factors such as fibromatosis gingivae.
- Delayed eruption of permanent tooth should be checked by radiographic examination, whether the teeth bud is present or absent. If present, the deciduous tooth needs to be extracted.
- In cases of ankylosed deciduous teeth, the ankylosed tooth should be surgically removed to prevent development of malocclusion, dental caries or local periodontal diseases.
- Behavior management techniques vary with the adults and children.
- The drug dosage differs for children and adults. The child dose can be calculated by the following formulas:
  Clark's rule: Child's age at next birthday/24 × Adult dose
  Young's rule: Child's age/Age + 12 × Adult dose
  Dilling rule: Age × Adult dose/20

Sex: Certain diseases show female predominance, whereas some others show, male predominance, such as dental caries due to more access to sweets, as their permanent teeth erupt at an early age (11–13 years) compared to males (14–16 years), so more exposure, female hormones, alteration in the composition of saliva and reduced flow during and more craving for food during pregnancy. Also females are more conscious of their esthetics when compared to males. Females are victims of sexual abuse and are also very sensitive and emotional. Thus dentists need to be careful with female patients.

Outpatient department number and date: A unique outpatient department (OPD) number or registration number should be given to each patient, which helps in identifying the patient and maintaining records at the dental office. This helps to know the details of the patient and the treatment done when the patient revisits.

Occupation: Enquire about working conditions as this may be very important if there is suspicion of exposure to an occupational hazard **(Table 1)**. Patients may attribute symptoms to work conditions, e.g. a headache from working in front of a computer screen. Other problems such as depression, chronic fatigue syndrome and general malaise may also be blamed on working conditions. Frequent job changes or chronic unemployment may reflect both socioeconomic circumstances and the patient's personality. Expensive treatments cannot be given to patients of low socioeconomic status. It is useful to enquire about specific stress in the workplace, such as bullying or the fear

Table 1: Occupational hazards

Occupational disease
• *Asbestos workers, builders:* Asbestosis, mesothelioma, attrition • *Coal miners:* Coal worker's pneumoconiosis • *Gold, copper, silicon and tin miners:* Pulmonary silicosis, attrition, erosion • *Farmers, vets, abattoir workers:* Brucellosis • *Aniline dye workers:* Bladder cancer • *Health care professionals:* Hepatitis B • *Carpenters, tailors, shoemakers:* Abrasion • *Lead, bismuth or cadmium factories:* Gingival staining • *Fisherman:* Cheilitis glandularis, carcinoma of lip

Table 2: Travel-related risks

Travel-related risks	
Viral diseases • Hepatitis A, B and C • Yellow fever • Rabies • Polio **Parasite and protozoan diseases** • Malaria • Schistosomiasis • Trypanosomiasis • Amoebiasis	**Bacterial diseases** • *Salmonella* • *Shigella* • Enteropathogenic *Escherichia coli* • Cholera • Meningitis • Tetanus • Lyme disease

of unemployment. Certain conditions have strong relationships to depression; however, limitation of lifestyle (work or social) may result in some more subtle negative effects on mood. Ask the patient about their mood to open up this line of enquiry. Chronic long-term stress may induce periodontal destruction.

Certain patients are related to such occupations where they have to travel often **(Table 2)**. In such cases, ask the patient about recent foreign travel. If so, determine the countries visited and, if the patient has returned from an area where malaria is endemic, ask about adequate prophylaxis for the appropriate period.

Education: Enquire about the age at which the patient left school and whether they attained any form of higher education or vocational skill. In addition, to providing useful background information, this information provides a context for assessing diseases and disorders causing intellectual deterioration and social function. This will also help in determining the level of awareness regarding oral diseases.

Address: Patient's address reveals the locality where they live, which may be helpful in identifying conditions, common eating habits, locality and surroundings. This helps in identifying the common conditions that are prevalent in that particular region, such as fluorosis, eating habits may inform us about the sugar consumption which in turn will aid in knowing the prevalence of caries.

Martial status: The martial status of patient/individual may be related to the stress associated with married individuals due to family pressure and consequent increased load due to other circumstances. However, stress may be a factor in patients who are single due to social pressure and work related pressure. The number of children that the patient has and their ages also should be taken into account.

Chief Complaint

Ask why the patient has come for advice; the 'chief complaint' (CC). There are a number of ways of approaching this; however, 'Why are you here?' can sound rude. Phrases such as 'What problem has brought you here today?', 'What is troubling you at the moment?' may be more appropriate. It is symptom/symptoms in patient's own words relating to presence of abnormal condition. It indicates the special reason why the patient seeks health care. Chief complaint should be recorded in the patient's own words because the complaints expressed as symptoms leave no room for doubt regarding patient's problem. Patients may have present with numerous complaints. This presents a problem to the clinical student who will list them all. For patients with lists of multiple problems, refine your history in the following ways:

- All the complaints that a patient identifies must be listed with the major problem listed first. Taking the history in chronological order is important. Describe how the symptom first began. What happened next? In addition, duration of the complaint should be added.
- Learn those symptoms that indicate a serious disease process is going on. If you know these symptoms, you can concentrate on them.
- Define what the major symptoms are, that is, what the patient feels. It is these troublesome symptoms that reduce a patient's quality of life the most.

If a patient uses a medical term, ask them what they mean, as sometimes their understanding is different to yours. Asking a patient to point to the affected area is often useful. Establish if the symptoms are improving, deteriorating or unchanged. Common chief complaints related to oral diseases are:

- Pain
- Loose teeth
- Bleeding
- Halitosis
- Swelling
- Sores
- Burning sensation
- Delayed tooth eruption
- Dry mouth
- Excessive salivation
- Paresthesia/Numbness

Pain in the teeth, mouth, face or head usually has a local cause; often the sequela of dental caries (odontogenic pain) but, there is the possibility of other disorders causing the pain **(Table 3)**. The real significance to the patient of orofacial pain can range from the benign to potentially lethal conditions. Some orofacial pain or headaches have an obvious but relatively unimportant cause (e.g. a hangover). Others have no obvious underlying organic pathology (e.g. atypical facial pain); some can threaten sight (e.g. giant cell arteritis or benign intracranial hypertension); whereas yet others can be life-threatening organic disorders (e.g. subarachnoid hemorrhage, bacterial meningitis, or brain tumors).

Table 3: Causes of orofacial pain

Local disorders	• Teeth, jaws and supporting tissues, maxillary sinus, salivary glands, pharynx and eyes
Neurological disorders	• Idiopathic trigeminal neuralgia • Malignant neoplasms involving the trigeminal nerve • Glossopharyngeal neuralgia • Herpes zoster (including postherpetic neuralgia) • Multiple sclerosis
Possible psychogenic causes	• Atypical facial pain • Burning mouth syndrome • Temporomandibular pain-dysfunction
Vascular disorders	• Migraine, migrainous neuralgia and giant cell arteritis
Referred pain	• Nasopharyngeal, ocular or aural • Cardiorespiratory: Angina • Lesions in the neck or chest (including lung cancer)

History of Present Illness

It is the record of narrative account of patient's problem from the onset to present time listing all the symptoms, signs and treatment undergone, if any in a chronological order. Once you have established the presenting complaint(s), identify the precise details of the current problem(s): the 'history of the presenting illness' (HOPI). Direct and specific questions are used to elicit the required information and can be recorded in narrative form as follows:

a. When did the problem start? and what did you notice first?
b. What makes the problem worse or better and have the symptoms become worse or better any time?
c. Any postural or diurnal (related to morning/evening time) variations?
d. Did you have any other problems or symptoms associated with this?
e. Any previous history of the same type?
f. Have you consulted any dentist or physician regarding the complaint?
g. Any treatment taken before or any medication being taken now and when did treatment start?

With pain problems history becomes more critical since it may be the only source of diagnostic information available. A well-described acronym, SOCRATES, is best used to elicit the features of pain; however, it is useful for many symptoms.

SOCRATES: The features of the history of the presenting complaint
Site: Where is the pain? And whether it is localized, diffuse or radiating? *Onset:* When did pain first begin? *Character (Nature):* Dull, piercing, throbbing, pulsating or burning? *Radiation and manner of flow of pain:* Steady or paroxysmal? *Associated features:* Lacrimation, nasal congestion or flushing. *Timing:* How often does it occur? Is the pain constant, intermittent, recurrent or momentary? *Exacerbating or alleviating features:* Does anything trigger it? Face movements, jaw movements, tongue movements, swelling, tensions or type of food consumed. *Severity:* Mild, moderate, severe or excruciating?

It is difficult to assess pain severity. Offering a patient a numerical score for pain, from '0' for no pain to '10' for excruciating pain, may provide a quantitative assessment of the symptom. So, each symptom should be expanded by detailed enquiry concerning development and relation to other symptoms. A comprehensive and valuable write up of the present illness necessitates a good basic knowledge of diseases of oral cavity so the interviewer is able to trace out leads given by a patient during interview.

Past Dental History

It provides information about the various episodes of illness, its treatment and patient's response. The information gathered may or may not be significant in regard to patient's chief complaint but it can provide with patient's back ground and must always be reviewed. Past dental history provides us the basis to evaluate the patient's current dental status and how the patient will respond to the proposed treatment.

Following are the details that should be investigated:

- Frequency of visits to dentist.
- Past experience during and after local anesthesia.
- Past experience during and after extraction.
- Past periodontal therapy, orthodontic treatment, dental appliance history, restorations or root canal fillings.
- Any surgical procedures besides extraction.
- Complications, if any.

Past Medical History

Why ask about past problems, illnesses and surgery? The past medical history (PMH) of a patient is incredibly important for ascertaining whether the patient is generally fit and well. Patients recall their medical history with varying degrees of detail and accuracy. Some provide a detailed history, whilst others need reminding. You can jog a patient's memory by asking if they have ever been admitted to hospital or undergone a surgical procedure, including cesarean sections in women. Certain conditions are often not volunteered or remembered when you ask, for example, high blood pressure (hypertension), ischemic heart disease (heart attacks, angina), high cholesterol (hypercholesterolemia), diabetes, epilepsy, asthma or other chest/lung/breathing problems, cancer, rheumatic fever and tuberculosis. Ask about these conditions specifically. Also included are any chronic childhood illnesses such as measles, rubella, mumps, whooping cough, chickenpox, rheumatic fever, scarlet fever, and polio. If the patient mentions specific illnesses or diagnoses, explore them in more detail. For example, if a patient mentions asthma, ask for a full description of the attacks so that you can decide whether or not the label is correct. Various questions may be required to obtain this information:

- Have you had any major illnesses in the past?
- Is there anything you regularly go to your physician for?
- Have you ever been into hospital before?
- Are you on any medication for X?

When taking the history of a child, it is usual to ask questions about the presence of any problems during pregnancy and birth, and about the progression of development. Learn the important developmental milestones of young children. Immunization history (or lack of it), growth and nutrition are all important in a pediatric history (if not immunized write down the reasons).

Past medical history (PMH) serves to establish a relationship between oral diseases and past systemic problems and consists of previously known and established medical facts. Primary function of this history is to avoid complications during dental treatment.

Past medical history (PMH) is usually organized in following sub-divisions:

- Any serious illnesses
- Hospitalizations
- Blood transfusions
- Allergies/immunizations
- Menstrual/pregnancy/menopause
- Medications
- Reviews of symptoms of systemic diseases of importance to the dentist
- Accidents/injuries

Cardiovascular System

The cardiovascular history is obtained to identify evidence of organic heart disease or symptoms that suggest the presence, or possible presence, of cardiovascular abnormalities. A search for cardiac risk factors is also appropriately incorporated into the past history. Has the patient ever been told he or she has high or low blood sugar? (The latter is not a risk factor, but suggests that a blood glucose may have been drawn in the past). Has the patient had high cholesterol or triglycerides, or high or low blood pressure? Has the patient smoked, chewed tobacco, or used snuff in the past? What about parenteral drugs (legal or illegal)? Has the patient been overweight? A past history of cardiovascular disease is an extremely important part of the patient's evaluation and should not be dismissed as noncontributory.

Has the patient ever had, or been told he or she had, a heart problem? If so, what? Taking a cardiac history involves checking that all components of the heart work. Dysfunction of any of these presents in the following manner:

- Reduced blood supply presents with chest pain or discomfort (often like a band or tightness) which may move or radiate into the neck, jaw, shoulder or left arm. The pain may come on with a fixed amount of exercise (stable angina) or suddenly at rest (suggesting a critical ischemia or acute coronary syndrome).
- An inefficient pump causes an accumulation of fluid and reduced output. Left heart failure results in fluid gathering in the lungs so the person may present with dyspnea (shortness of breath) or shortness of breath lying flat (orthopnea). To compensate for this positional problem it is often useful to ask patients how many pillows they sleep with. Right heart failure results in fluid gathering in the lower limbs (peripheral edema) or sacrum (sacral edema) and in the neck veins.
- Patients with pump failure may have a very limited exercise tolerance.
- Electrical disturbances may result in a feeling of palpitations (an awareness of the heart beating) which may be fast or slow, regular or irregular. The patient might be able to tap out the rhythm. Other disturbances may result in dizziness, light-headedness or collapse as not enough blood reaches the brain.
- Valve problems may result in sudden collapse, weakness/light-headedness or dizziness or reduced exercise tolerance.
- If the lower limb arteries are involved in atherosclerosis the patient may complain of intermittent claudication or they may have pale, cold, painful toes and feet, leg ulcers or ischemic toes. Atherosclerosis affecting the carotid arteries may cause a stroke (facial droop, weakness or slurred speech), a transient neurological deficit or loss of vision. Carotid artery calcification may be detected during routine orthopantomograms (OPG's) used for radiographic evaluation and may aid in identifying this life-threatening condition in affected individuals.

Obtain details regarding the diagnosis, when it was made, who made it, how it was diagnosed, and what was done about it. Ask questions such as:

- Did you have any operations of chest, heart valves in childhood? This indicates septal defects or presence of pacemaker.
- Did you suffer from fleeting joint pains, sore throat or fever? This indicates rheumatic fever which requires antibiotic prophylaxis during dental treatment to prevent the occurrence of sub acute bacterial endocarditis (SABE).
- Do you have any breathlessness on exertion? This would point towards congestive cardiac failure (CCF) which may be the cause of dry mouth due the side effects of digitalis and diuretics that are being administered.
- Do you have pain on left side of chest? This may point that the patient may have angina. Sublingual nitroglycerine is administered to these patients during the attack. If the patients do not respond it may lead to myocardial infarction. These patients may have a high caries rate as the binder of nitroglycerine is cariogenic.

- Do you have high blood pressure? Such patients present with complications during dental procedures, due to the effect of anticoagulant therapy.
- Ever got a stroke?

Respiratory System

Sometimes damage to the respiratory center in the brainstem or medication will reduce the respiratory rate. The respiratory rate can increase in the absence of lung disease (if the patient is shocked or acidotic). Important respiratory findings include chest pain, wheeze, cough, sputum, hoarseness, shortness of breath (when and relieving factors), cyanosis and exercise tolerance. Following questions may be asked:

- Do you have any sort of breathing problems? Breathing difficulties may arise because of:
  - *Infection:* Localized or generalized.
  - *Airway narrowing:* Either reversible (asthma or bronchospasm) or obstructive (COPD).
  - Airway disease that results in either thickening/fibrosis of the airways, destruction of the small airway (bullous disease) or lung collapse (pneumothorax).
  - Reduced blood supply.
  - Trauma.
- Do you have problems of wheezing? This may be due to:
  - Asthma
  - Chronic obstructive pulmonary diseases
  - Pneumonia
  - Acute bronchitis.

  Dental treatment for asthmatic patients needs to address oral manifestations of this condition. Oral manifestations are decreased salivary flow, increased calculus, increased gingivitis, increased periodontal diseases and increased incidence of caries.

  In the asthmatic patients, fluoride supplements should be instituted, patient should be instructed to rinse his mouth after using inhalers. In such patients use stress reducing techniques, have oxygen and bronchodilators available, care should be taken in positioning the suction tips and judicious use of rubber dams.
- Did you get swelling of ankles or legs? This may point towards COPD.

Gastrointestinal System

The history of past gastrointestinal diseases encompasses disorders of the esophagus, stomach, pancreas, gallbladder, and biliary tract, as well as jaundice. Important symptoms include nausea, vomiting, appetite, difficulties in swallowing (liquid, solid), weight loss (intentional), diarrhea (mucous, blood), constipation, steatorrhea (fatty stools that do not flush away), change in bowel habit, ulcers (mouth, stomach, intestine) and jaundice. Following questions should be asked to the patient:

- Do you have heart burn/acidity/foul taste?
- Do you have bouts of nausea, lack of appetite?
- Did you suffer from jaundice/hepatitis?

Endocrine System

Most endocrine disorders do not present as a single visible or palpable abnormality. Physical diagnoses rely on astute observations by the examiner, who, after a careful history, has some clue as to the diagnosis. Endocrine diagnosis involves the sequence of history, physical examination, laboratory, and radiologic evaluation. A patient with one endocrine disease (e.g. Hashimoto's thyroiditis) is at greater risk for the development of other endocrine disorders (e.g. adrenal, testicular, or ovarian failure). A patient may harbor more than one endocrinopathy, which could be overlooked if subtle historical and clinical clues are not heeded. Severe endocrinopathies may influence the treatment of dental patients. Those tend to precipitate acute problems are hyperthyroidism, diabetes mellitus, Addison's disease and steroid therapy. The important signs include thyroid trouble, heat or cold intolerance, excessive sweating, excessive thirst or hunger, polyuria, change in glove or shoe size. Following questions should be asked to identify the underlying endocrinopathy:

- Do you have excessive thirst/hunger/frequent urination? This indicates that the patient is diabetic.
- Do you have sudden loss of weight and tremors of hands? It is suggestive of hyperthyroidism. In cases of thyrotoxicosis due to infection or surgery, it may lead to thyroid storm, which may precipitate a heart attack. Dental treatment should be postponed and rapid control of oral infection is essential in this condition.
- Are you on steroid therapy? Such patients may present with inability to respond to stress. Prolonged use of steroids may lead to delayed wound healing, osteoporosis and capillary fragility.

Hematopoietic

Hematological diseases involve the red blood cells, the granulocytes, the lymphocytes and monocytes of the immune system, and the platelets and the clotting proteins of the hemostatic system. Manifestations of any kind of blood dyscrasias may be seen in oral cavity. Dentist must know limitations on dental treatment imposed by blood dyscrasias, such as anemic patients are susceptible to shock and may experience difficulty during stressful conditions. Any history of prolonged bleeding and easy bruising may indicate towards hemophilia/purpura. A careful search for lymph nodes in all the lymph node bearing areas of the body must be made in the patient with leukemia or lymphoma as well as palpation for splenomegaly or hepatomegaly.

Musculoskeletal System

The patient may complain of pain, reduced movement, loss of function, numbness or altered sensation. Acutely inflamed joints (either from a bursa, an inflammatory arthritis or joint infection) may present with red (erythema), hot, swollen, tender joints that they have difficulty moving. The important signs that should be examined include weakness, pain, stiffness (when and duration), fractures, ability to dress self-completely, ability to walk-up and down stairs. The following questions may be asked:

- Has the patient experienced bone or joint pain?
- Has joint pain been accompanied by swelling, tenderness or redness?
- Is the pain confined to a single joint or is it more diffuse?
- Does the pain predominate on walking or does it appear as the relevant joint is used (e.g. in walking)?
- Is there a history of trauma to the affected joint and is there a family history of joint disease?

Patient's mobility or ability to move major parts of the body is carefully observed. Healthy persons will move all their limbs, head and neck with smooth easy movements. Patients with rheumatoid arthritis/osteoarthritis will have greatly decreased mobility of arms, legs and fingers. Hyperelasticity/hyperextensibility of joints is observed in Marfan's Syndrome and Ehler-Danlos Syndrome. Fleeting joint pains are observed in rheumatic fever. Small peripheral joints are observed in gout and rheumatoid arthritis.

Neurologic System

The brain tissue does not perceive pain well so disorders within the brain can present with pain due to stretching or irritation of the meninges or a loss of normal brain function. Patients may complain of headaches, faints, fits, loss of function, loss of sensation/altered sensation, visual disturbance, nausea or vomiting, limb (paralysis or paraparesis) and facial weakness, strokes, abnormal behavior and hallucinations (visual suggest organic disease, olfactory suggest epilepsy, auditory suggest psychiatric disease).

The peripheral nervous system may also be damaged at the level of the spinal cord or along the peripheral nerve itself. Autonomic dysfunction often presents with loss of sympathetic function so the person may not be able to regulate their heart rate, blood pressure or skin temperature appropriately. Damage to the peripheral nerve may result in abnormal sensation (paresthesia) or partial or complete loss of function (paralysis or palsy). Such patients may be needed to handle with appropriate care and precautions. Stress during dental procedures must be minimized. These patients may also present with poor oral hygiene due to abnormal motor functions and loss of sensation due to paralysis or paresthesia.

Cranial Nerve Examination

It is important to evaluate whether there is any cranial nerve dysfunction that might relate to patient's oral symptoms. An answer to this question usually comes from specific testing of cranial nerve function as a part of routine general clinical examination.

Olfactory nerve: Its functioning can be evaluated by one of the nostrils of the patient and asking him to smell nonirritating substances, i.e. tea, coffee, clove oil, peppermint oil from other nostril. Disorders can be evaluated as:

No smell: Anosmia
Perversion of smell: Parosmia
Unpleasant odor: Cacosmia

Optic nerve: Optic nerve function is tested by investigation of visual acuity, visual field and color vision.

Visual acuity is measured by finger counting at a distance of 1 m it can also be tested using Snellens' test types with series of letters of varying sizes. Top letters are visible at distance of 60 m, with consecutive lines at distance of 36 m, 24 m, 18 m, 12 m, 9 m, 6 m and 5 m.

VA = d/D

Where, d = distance at which letters are read and D = distance at which letters should be read.

Jaggers' chart is used to measure visual acuity for near vision.

Visual field can be measured by confrontation test and color vision is tested by pseudo isochromatic plates of Ishihara.

Oculomotor, trochlear and abducent nerves: These are responsible for the movements of the eyeball and hence if affected singly/together, they cause defective ocular movements. III, IV and VI cranial nerves are listed simultaneously by examining size, outline, reaction of each pupil to light and dark and to accommodation for near and far vision. Conjugate eye movements, individual eye movements, convergent vision are all tested by asking the patient to follow the path of pencil held at a distance and close up, as it traverses right to left and up and down movements.

Paralysis of oculomotor nerve is characterized by eyeballs deviated laterally and downwards; difficulty in reading, asymmetrical pupils (Aniscoria), ptosis, loss of papillary vasoconstrictor function, diplopia and squint.

Paralysis of trochlear nerve shows upwards and inwards deviated eyeballs.

Paralysis of abducent nerve demonstrates medially deviated eyeballs.

Trigeminal nerve: This nerve is tested for both motor and sensory function. Motor function is tested by asking the patient to clench his teeth, normally masseter and temporalis stand out in equal prominence, tested by palpating the muscles. Lateral movement of the jaw against the examiner finger is one test of pterygoid function and patient is asked to open the mouth. Jaw deviates to healthy side being pushed by lateral pterygoid muscle.

Jaw jerk: Abnormalities of the jaw jerk may indicate muscular weakness or an abnormality of proprioceptive reflex arc controlling jaw movements. The index finger is pressed downward and posteriorly above the mental eminence, and lightly striked with percussion hammer/finger. In normal subjects, a single reflex response can usually be discerned by palpation.

Sensory function can be assessed by corneal reflex and by using instruments such as Graded Frey's Hair, two-point esthesiometers, calibrated thermal devices, discs of various grades of sand paper for the evaluation of textural differences, stereognostic forms for the evaluation of oral stereotactic ability and taste testing.

Facial nerve: Motor function is tested by observing facial muscle function in response to requests to wrinkle the forehead, frown, close the eyelids tightly, wink, open the mouth, puffing of cheeks, pucker the lips, whistle and speak. Close observation and comparison of right and left sides may be necessary to detect minor degrees of facial palsy. Gustatory function is tested by checking the flow of saliva following application of lemon juice or citric acid to the affected side of mouth.

Auditory nerve: Acoustic nerve function includes both hearing and vestibular components, which are physiologically distinct and tested separately. Auditory function tested by Rinne's test (vibrating fork in front of ear and then on mastoid bone) and Weber's test (vibrating tuning fork kept in middle of forehead and vibrations heard in both the ears). Vestibular function is assessed by employing the rotational tests to produce changes in endolymph current in semicircular canals which produces nausea, vertigo, dizziness and horizontal nystagmus when vestibular status is intact.

Glossopharyngeal, vagus nerve: These are tested together, as palate fails to elevate to close off the nasopharynx there is nasal quality to speech, dysphagia, and nasal regurgitation of liquids. Observe the symmetry in elevation of palate and uvula with drooping of palatal arch on affected side and median raphe moving towards the unaffected side. Swallowing and cough reflex is served by 9th and 10th cranial nerves, dysfunctioning leads to dysarthria and drooling of saliva. Pharyngeal component of the vagus nerve can be tested by Gag reflex and laryngeal component can be studied by inspection of laryngeal function with indirect laryngoscopy.

Accessory nerve: It is tested through its motor supply to the trapezius and sternomastoid muscles. For trapezius, ask the patient to shrug his shoulders against the resistance to examiner hands; for the sternomastoid muscle, have the patient turn and flex the head against the resistance.

Hypoglossal nerve: This nerve supplies motor supply to tongue; paralysis causes deviation of the tongue when the patient extrudes it. Lesion above the hypoglossal nucleus to peripheral nerves causes atrophy and fasciculations on the tongue. Bilateral lesions lead to dysarthria, difficulty in swallowing and inability to protrude tongue.

Genitourinary

Pain in the abdominal wall just under the lower ribs area can suggest renal injury. Dull, constant pain suggests infection, bruising or a possible blockage in urine flow resulting in dilatation of the renal pelvis (hydronephrosis). Sharp, intermittent, severe (colicky) pain radiating from loin to groin that causes the patient to move around is suggestive of a renal calculus (stone). Ask about any veneral diseases such as syphilis, which may be the cause of the congenital syndrome characterized by Hutchinson incisors, mulberry molars and altered 8th cranial nerve function.

Hospitalization, if any: To determine possible history of an illness that may be defined as serious, resulting in hospitalization of the patient, it is necessary to ask about previous hospitalization of the patient. It is necessary to enquire the further information regarding the cause, length of time of hospitalization. Patients should also be inquired about whether they ever had an operation and what procedure was carried out? History regarding the use of local and general anesthesia, complications with the anesthetic and healing of the surgical wound should also be recorded.

Blood Transfusions

Questions regarding blood transfusions may uncover the blood dyscrasias or other conditions. The patients should be asked about the quantity, cause, frequency and complications, if any associated with blood transfusions.

Allergies

Establishing if a patient has ever had an adverse reaction to a medication is important. This is a crucial step that must be documented before any drugs are prescribed. Sometimes it is difficult to differentiate if the patient had an allergic reaction or whether the reaction was a recognized side effect of the treatment. A severe allergic reaction or anaphylactic reaction includes facial swelling, especially of the mouth and throat, bronchospasm and respiratory distress, hemodynamic shock and reduced level of consciousness. The reaction to the following medication should be noted:

- Aspirin/NSAID's
- Penicillin
- Sulfonamides (Sulfa drugs)
- Cumarin derivatives
- Local anesthesia
- Barbiturates
- *Analgesics:* Opioids

Also enquire about any other allergies due to certain food stuffs, pollen grains, dust or other agents.

Pregnancy

Important obstetric questions include: number of pregnancies, miscarriages or terminations. Also ask about previous obstetric complications or surgery. If the patient is pregnant, ask about the current trimester, since dental treatment is most safe to be done in the second trimester. It is avoided in the first trimester as during this organogenesis takes place and inadvertent exposure to radiation or certain drugs may lead to unforeseen congenital defects in the newborn. There may be risk of premature delivery due to the stress induced during dental treatment in the third trimester; hence treatment is avoided during the third trimester. Care should be taken in pregnant females to avoid excessive exposure to radiations, use of lead aprons and avoid use of certain drugs like Tetracycline/Thalidomide.

Medications

The patient's drug history includes past and present medications, recreational drugs and adverse effects of medications. Patients often think that you only need to know about prescription medication so do remember to ask about over-the-counter medication, alternative treatments and recreational drug use. Many patients do not know the names of their medication and it is useful to ask for the labeled bottles or a written prescription. It is important to recognize some medications and ask about them, specifically, medications that increase the risk of bleeding, that alter vital signs or reduce consciousness and those that are dangerous if taken in excess. Examples of these include; warfarin, aspirin and clopidogrel increase bleeding, β blockers reduce heart rate, opiates, e.g. codeine or morphine and benzodiazepines, e.g. diazepam, temazepam can reduce consciousness and drugs that are dangerous in excess include digoxin, lithium and theophyllines. Remember to ask about nonprescription medicines, herbal and alternative remedies since some of them interact with commonly used medications.

Past medications may have caused an allergic reaction or were ineffective. Either way, you need to make sure the patient is not put back on that medication. Make a list of the medications the patient is on and ask how long they have been on each one (is this the cause of the presenting complaint? For example phenytoin induced gingival hyperplasia). Remember that iatrogenic disease is very common and always consider drug-related side-effects in the differential diagnosis. Ask women of reproductive age about their choice of contraceptive and postmenopausal women about hormone replacement therapy.

Family History

The family history may reveal evidence of an inherited disorder **(Table 4)**. Information about the immediate family may also have considerable bearing on the patient's symptoms. Social partnerships, marriage, sexual orientation and close emotional attachments are complex systems which exert profound influences on health and illness. A useful starting point might be to ask if the patient has a regular partner or is married. If so, ask about their health status or any recent change in health status. If the patient has children, determine their ages and state of health. When there is suspicion of a familial disorder, it is helpful to construct a family tree. Outline the age and health, or age and cause of death, of each immediate relative, including parents, grandparents, siblings, children, and grandchildren. Enquire whether any near relatives died in childhood and if so, from what cause. If the pattern of inheritance suggests a recessive trait, ask whether the parents were related in particular whether they were first cousins.

Family history should include the most important conditions that follow familial pattern. Moreover, it also identifies possible exposure to communicable diseases that may involve the patient. Equally important is information in regard to dental status of parents and siblings. This helps to reveal genetic makeup of patient's dentition. Just as with families, interactions with wider society can exert powerful influences on health and well-being. A detailed social history includes enquiries about schooling, past and present employment, social support networks, and leisure.

Table 4: Common diseases expressed in families
• Hyperlipidemia (ischemic heart disease) • Diabetes mellitus • Hypertension • Hemophilia • Myopia • Migraine • Neurologic diseases • Alcoholism • Depression • Osteoporosis • Cancer (Bowel, ovarian, breast)

Personal History

Dentist should attempt to gain insight into personal habits and habits related to the oral cavity. This information may be important in determining the prognosis. It is also convenient to ask about the use of tobacco and alcohol: the quantity smoked and the number of units drunk each week.

Tobacco Consumption

Patients usually give a fairly accurate account of their smoking. Ask what form of tobacco they consume and for how long they have been smoking. Ask about betel nut and pan chewing. If they previously smoked, when did they stop and for how long did they abstain? Many red and white, benign and malignant oral lesions are a result of tobacco consumption such as:

- Smoker's palate
- Reverse smoker's palate

- Sniff dipper lesion
- Smoker's lip lesions
- Oral submucous fibrosis
- Palatal erythema
- Hairy tongue
- Erythroplakia
- Oral lichen planus
- Squamous cell carcinoma.

Alcohol Consumption

Unlike smoking, alcohol history is often inaccurate with a tendency to underestimate intake. Many patients consider beer and wine to be less alcoholic than spirits. Establish the type of alcohol the patient consumes and assess their intake in units. If the patient is vague, ask how long a bottle of wine or spirits might last or the amount they drank over a specific recent time period (e.g. yesterday or over the last week). Alcohol-dependent patients often deny when questioned about alcohol consumption and a third party history from friends and family is often revealing and helpful. Certain questions may reveal dependency without asking the patient to specify consumption. Ask about early morning nausea, vomiting and tremulousness, which are typical features of dependency. Ask whether they ever drink alone, when they first wake up in the morning, or during the course of the day as well as in the evenings. Do they have alcohol-free days?

Alcohol consumption may cause certain central nervous system (CNS) disorders (withdrawal convulsions, alcoholic dementia, subdural hematoma, peripheral neuropathy, etc.), gastrointestinal (GI) diseases (peptic ulcers, pancreatitis, gastritis, esophagitis and Mallory-Weiss syndrome), cardiovascular system (CVS) related (cardiomyopathy and hypertension), liver related (cirrhosis, alcoholic hepatitis and stenosis) and genitourinary related (impotence, infertility and fetal alcoholic syndrome).

Habits Related to Oral Cavity

Ask questions about the method, frequency and material used for brushing the teeth. Also ask about the timing and method of cleaning, and whether the patient uses any other oral hygiene aids such as, floss, interdental brush or mouthwash. This helps to know about the patients' awareness towards maintaining oral hygiene and their level of education about various methods of cleaning and use of other aids.

Also ask about any habits related to the oral cavity such as tongue thrusting, cheek and lip biting, thumb sucking, bruxism, mouth breathing and nail biting. Identification of the habit may help to identify the underlying malocclusion, deep palate, swollen anterior gingiva, open bite, increased incidence of caries, mobility of teeth, temporomandibular joint pain, tenderness and hypertrophy of masticatory muscles and fractures of teeth and restorations in the individual with the associated habit.

Dietary Habit

Ask questions regarding the frequency, type of sugar (fermentable or non-fermentable and solid/liquid/sticky) and time (with meals or in between meals) of sugar consumption. Also ask about whether the patient is vegetarian or nonvegetarian. This helps us know about the increased caries prevalence in individuals with high consumption of sticky sugars in between meals.

Comprehensive and valuable write-up of case history elicits good basic knowledge of oral diseases so that interviewer is able to trace out leads given by patient during interview.

4

General Physical Examination of Patient

Introduction

Examination of the patient represents the second stage of diagnostic procedure and it is a clinician's contribution to the diagnostic procedure. An established routine is important because it minimizes the possibility of overlooking previously undiscovered/unknown lesions.

Physical examination is the process of evaluating objective anatomic findings through the use of the following principles:

Inspection: It is the most productive and frequently used examination technique. Inspection is a systematic visual assessment of patient under observation. It is defined as the observation with an unaided eye. Slight oversight may result in missed diagnosis. It should incorporate general observation and close detailed chair-side investigation.

Palpation: It is an act of feeling by sense of touch. It is a procedure where examiner feels or presses upon the structures or portions of the body. In order to realize maximum benefit from palpation, clinician must know normal gross anatomy, location of tissues/organs, their extent and their anatomic relationship to each other. Palpation can be bilateral, bimanual or bidigital.

Percussion: It is the act of striking a portion of body with fingers or an instrument to evaluate condition of underlying structures by careful attention to sound or echo produced. It aids in evaluating and localization of inflammation of periodontal ligament and secondary pulpitis, evaluating the character and density of supporting tissues and amount of alveolar bone surrounding the tooth and evaluating the muscle reflex.

Auscultation: It is the act of listening to the sounds produced within the body. This is one of the least appreciated facets of clinical examination. It aids in listening the sounds of abnormal breathing, clicking and snapping sounds of temporomandibular disorders (TMJ), vocal fremitus and other abnormalities, determination of relationship of oral structures to production of normal speech.

General physical examination of patient as a whole gives clues to the diagnosis. This begins the moment the patient steps in a clinic and is first observed. This is an art which has to be acquired after a good deal of experience. The information obtained must be thoughtfully integrated with the patient's history and pathophysiology. The physical examination, thoughtfully performed, should yield 20% of the data necessary for patient diagnosis and management. Information pertinent to the physical examination can be learned from observation of speech, gestures, habits, gait, and manipulation of features and extremities. Interactions with relatives and staff are often revealing. Pigmentary changes such as cyanosis, jaundice, and pallor may be noted. The physical examination, however, can be the weak link in this chain if it is performed in a perfunctory and superficial manner. Understanding the pathophysiologic mechanism of a physical abnormality is essential for correct diagnosis and management.

Objectives of general physical examination are as follows:
- Protection of the patient from the harm that might be caused by dental treatment.
- Protect the dentist and auxiliary staff from possible contiguous diseases.
- Dentist can serve as a case finder in suspecting early systemic disease problems.

General physical examination is done to record the following:

General Examination

Built and Nourishment

It is the skeletal structure in relation to age and sex of the individual as compared to normal person. It is calculated based on height to weight ratio.

Nourishment is the muscular development seen in the patient. A patient can be defined as well built or malnourished on the basis of nourishment. It is done by calculating the Basal Metabolic Rate. Certain clinical signs help to diagnose the deficiency of proteins, vitamins, fats, carbohydrates and minerals.

Body Build (Physique)

It can be of the following types based on:
- *Adipose tissue:* Esthetic (thin), plethoric (obese) and athletic (well-nourished).
- *According to Sheldon:* Ectomorphic (tall and thin), mesomorphic (average) and endomorphic (short and obese).
- *According to Kampmeier and Blake:* Sthenic, hyposthenic and hypersthenic.

Gait

Observe the patient the moment he enters the clinic, for any abnormality in the usual smooth movements in which they move. A classical example of abnormal gait is seen in tertiary syphilis in the form of Tabes dorsalis. Patient's gait is very unsteady because they search for ground at each step. Depressed patients often drag their feet, while ataxic patients have a shuffling gait. Pain can have a dramatic effect on a person's ability to move. Sometimes pain causes the patient to adopt a protective gait.

Thus, the presence of abnormal gait is diagnostic to introduce the examiner to the possibility of paralysis or other neuromuscular disorders that may have a dental correlation. Examiner must attempt to identify the areas that are involved since dental treatment many times will be dictated by the location and extent of paralysis.

Posture

Posture can be referred to the way the patient stands. Abnormal posture may be:

- *Kyphosis:* Posterior rounding of thoracic spine. It is congenital and is observed in tuberculosis, osteitis deformans or due to neurological disturbances.
- *Lordosis:* Anterior rounding of lumber spine. It is physiological and due to muscular dystrophy or large abdominal tumors.
- *Scoliosis:* Lateral curvature of spine. It is also congenital and may be due to neurological or functional causes or as a result of rickets.

Patients with degenerative arthritis/osteoporosis present with stooped spine and are frequently hump-backed. Patients with pain develop bent/stooped design to relieve some pain. Depressed patients have a drooping posture.

Height and Weight

They provide a clue to the growth and maturation of the patient that may have dentofacial correlation. Abnormal variations in height can be either gigantism or dwarfism. Gigantism may be simple or primary gigantism (racial, familial or constitutional), due to hyperpituitarism, hypergonadism, Marfan's syndrome, Klinefelter's syndrome, homocystinuria). Dwarfism may be genetic, due to Down's syndrome, Turner's syndrome, Noonan's syndrome, delayed puberty, malnourishment, malabsorption, rickets, hypopituitarism, hypothyroidism, Cushing's syndrome, excessive androgens, achondroplasia, congenital cyanotic heart disease, etc.

Acute weight gain around the abdomen is often due to one of the 5 F's: fat, fluid, feces, flatulence and fetus. A history may give further information on this. Fluid retention is often due to failure of the heart, liver or kidneys or in very low protein states. Weight loss is often not recognized by the patient. Clues include temporal wasting (a loss of the muscle at the side of the eyes, creating a hollow), a new notch on the belt or an increase in the amount of loose clothes. Severe weight loss is referred to as cachexia or the person is cachectic.

Vital Signs

Blood Pressure

The circulatory system is a closed system. When the heart contracts, a volume of blood is propelled into the arterial system and is measured as the systolic blood pressure (systole means cardiac contraction). During relaxation of the heart, the amount of constriction (or squeeze) applied to the arteries and the volume of blood in them is measured as the diastolic pressure. An instrument called a sphygmomanometer is used to measure blood pressure (BP). The aneroid gauge (or mercury column) is calibrated in even numbers. When measuring blood pressure, it is important to select the proper cuff. Cuffs those are too small for the patient may give falsely high readings. In addition, remember that cuffs should not be placed over heavy or tight clothing.

With the patient seated, and their arm resting comfortably on a level surface (the cuff should be at the same level as the heart), apply the cuff to the upper arm about 1 inch above the flexion crease at the elbow. Center the bladder of the cuff over the brachial artery (usually an arrow marked artery can be found on the cuff label). Palpate the medial aspect of the antecubital space to detect the pulsation in the brachial artery. Place the stethoscope in your ears with the earpieces pointing toward the front of your head.

Next, place the diaphragm side of the stethoscope over the spot you have located and inflate the cuff rapidly until sounds are no longer heard in the artery. Inflate the cuff 20 mm Hg beyond this point, and then gradually deflate the cuff while listening for tapping sounds in the artery. When the sounds are first heard regularly, this level is the systolic blood pressure. Note the reading on the gauge. Continue to deflate the cuff slowly. The character of the sounds will change and finally abruptly disappear; this is the diastolic blood pressure. Again, note the reading indicated on the gauge. With the test completed, fully open the valve to deflate the cuff and remove it from the patient's arm. The blood pressure is recorded on the patient's chart as the systolic pressure over the diastolic pressure and also indicates the arm in which it was taken. A slight variation in blood pressure can occur between the arms; this is normal. A typical chart notation might be: 120/80 arm.

Blood pressure classifications are shown in **Table 1**. Systolic pressures less than 20 mm Hg of the patient's normal reading may indicate hypotension. Since the diastolic pressure is the resting pressure of the heart, it is closely monitored for the development of hypertension. Several factors, including stress and anxiety, can raise the blood pressure and variations in blood pressure can be noted throughout the day. Before a diagnosis of hypertension is made, blood pressure should be taken on different days at different times.

Table 1: Joint National Commission (JNC-2003) VII BP classification

Category	*Systolic BP (mm Hg)*	*Diastolic BP (mm Hg)*
Normal	<120	<80
Prehypertensive	120–139	80–89
Stage I	140–159	90–99
Stage II	≥160	≥100
Stage III	≥180	≥110

Pulse

The pulse is the pressure wave that can be felt as the heart contracts and propels a volume of blood forward in the arterial system. For routine measurement, the pulse in the radial artery in the wrist is most commonly used, which can be palpated on the thumb side of the anterior aspect of the wrist. Apply gentle pressure to the artery until the pulsations can be felt. 2 or 3 fingers should be used to assess the pulse. The thumb should be avoided as you may be feeling (and counting) your own pulse rate and not that of the patient.

The rate, strength, and regularity of the pulse can be assessed and should be recorded on the patient's chart. For adults and children above 10 years of age, the pulse is usually in the range of 60–100 beats/minute. For children of age below 1 year it ranges from 100 to 160 beats/minute and for children of 1–10 years age group the pulse ranges from 60 to 140 beats/minute. Well-trained athletes have a pulse of 40–60 beats/minute. Variations from this range are common. In adults, a pulse exceeding 100 beats/minute is termed tachycardia and bradycardia if it is less than 60 beats/minute. A person who exercises or runs regularly may normally have a resting heart rate less than 60, while a patient anxious about dental treatment may have a rapid pulse. Retaking the pulse in a few minutes often results in a more accurate value.

The strength of the pulse is a rough measurement of the amount of blood ejected by the heart and the amount of constriction in blood vessels. A weak, thready (small) pulse is an indication of shock and low blood pressure, while a bounding (strong) pulse is an indication of anxiety or high blood pressure. Regularity is indicated by even spacing between the beats. An irregular pulse, which indicates a rhythm disturbance of the heart, is seen in some patients and is usually not severe. In hypotensive or unresponsive patients, the carotid artery should be used to check for the presence of a pulse.

Respiratory Rate

The respiratory rate is determined by the number of breaths in 6 or 15 seconds. One breath or respiratory cycle consists of one inhalation and one exhalation. In many cases, if a patient knows someone is counting their respirations, he or she will unconsciously alter them. One easy method to measure the respiratory rate is to begin counting the rise and fall of the patient's chest immediately after taking their blood pressure or pulse. With the stethoscope still in your ears, glance at the clock, shift your gaze toward the patient's chest and begin counting. To obtain the respiratory rate, multiply the number of breaths in six seconds times ten (or the number of breaths in fifteen seconds times four). A normal respiratory rate for an adult at rest is between twelve and twenty times per minute. Factors that can increase the respiratory rate include anxiety, fever, and hypoxia. Respiratory rates can increase with age due to decreasing lung elasticity. The respiratory rate will decrease with the use of narcotics, including Demerol and morphine, as well as with the use of the benzodiazepines such as Valium. Note the rate, depth, and regularity of respirations, e.g. 16 normal and regular.

Temperature

Taking a temperature as part of the vitals check will often indicate if the patient has an infection. An oral temperature in excess of 99.6°F (37.5°C) is a good indicator of the presence of a viral or bacterial infection. The other vitals can be recorded while the thermometer is in the patient's mouth, thus using little additional chair time. Body temperature varies with location, and may be measured where most convenient. It can be measured from the tympanic, rectal or axillary location other than the oral cavity. In the dental office, the oral reading is most frequently used. The four most common types of thermometers include:

1. Digital oral thermometer, used with plastic probe covers.
2. Tympanic (ear) thermometers give a reading equivalent to the oral temperature.
3. Disposable thermometer tapes.
4. Standard glass thermometer with a mercury column inside, used with plastic probe covers.

Digital thermometers are popular due to their convenience and fast reading. The battery must be checked regularly for proper use and accurate readings. The digital reading is displayed on a small LCD screen after approximately 30 seconds.

A tympanic thermometer registers the body's temperature by bouncing an infrared signal off the eardrum. The reading is accurate and received within a few seconds. Disposable thermometer tapes or strips can be used orally or axially. The strips are convenient but will give inaccurate readings if improperly stored near a heat source. To receive a reading, the strip is placed in the mouth or against the forehead and the liquid crystals change color to indicate temperature.

The standard glass thermometer is the least expensive and may be calibrated in either degrees Fahrenheit or degrees Centigrade. These thermometers use mercury inside the glass cylinder to measure the temperature. Many states have banned their use because if broken, exposure to toxic mercury vapors can occur. Before taking the patient's temperature, the mercury should be shaken down to give a reading below 95°F. Shake the thermometer with a snapping downward motion, but take care to avoid striking it against a counter top or cabinet. If a glass thermometer is accidentally broken, a mercury clean-up kit should be used to prevent contamination. For this reason many offices are choosing to use thermometers without mercury.

Signs of Anemia

Anemia is defined as a decrease in the red blood cell mass. The World Health Organization has decided that anemia exists in adults whose hemoglobin values are lower than 13 g/dL in males and 12 g/dL in females. Children age 6 months to 6 years are considered anemic at hemoglobin levels below 11 g/dL; and between 6 and 14 years, below 12 g/dL.

An appearance of underdevelopment, malnutrition, or chronic illness, can be important clues to the underlying etiology of disease. Second, the skin and mucous membranes are pallor, show abnormal pigmentation, icterus, spider nevi, petechiae, purpura, angiomas, ulcerations, palmar erythema, coarseness of hair, puffiness of the face, thinning of the lateral aspects of the eyebrows, nail defects, and an unusual prominent venous pattern on the abdominal wall. The conjunctiva and sclera, can show pallor, icterus, splinter hemorrhages and petechiae.

Signs of Cyanosis

Cyanosis is a bluish color of mucous membranes and/or skin. While this is most frequently attributable to increased amounts of unoxygenated hemoglobin (deoxyhemoglobin) in the vasculature, there are other causes of bluish skin color.

When looking for cyanosis, one should inspect those body sites that contain minimal melanotic pigment, that have a capillary bed close to the skin surface, and that are well-perfused. Lips, ears, trunk, nailbed, hands, conjunctiva, and circumoral areas have been compared in detecting cyanosis due to arterial hypoxemia; the tongue is the most sensitive area, but the lips are more specific.

Central cyanosis is caused by direct shunting of venous blood into arterial side without being oxygenated in the lungs. It is observed due to congenital heart disease, pulmonary edema, bronchial asthma, emphysema, bronchopneumonia, pneumothorax, upper respiratory obstruction and due to higher altitude.

The usual pattern of cyanosis noted in conditions of reduced blood flow is for peripheral sites, in particular the extremities, to be affected preferentially (acrocyanosis). Central portions of the body are typically spared. Low flow may result from decreased arterial perfusion caused by poor cardiac output (as in cardiogenic shock), by fixed arterial narrowing (as in atherosclerosis), or by reflex arteriolar narrowing (as in cold weather). Venous obstruction slows capillary blood flow and may be caused by local (venous thrombosis) or central (congestive heart failure) mechanisms.

Eyes

The sclera (white area) of the eye maybe discolored; yellow discoloration suggests jaundice while redness may suggest local eye trauma or a systemic inflammatory condition. An increase in the number of red capillaries across the eye (conjunctival injection), associated with a film of water over the eyes (chemosis), like a tear that does not fall suggest carbon dioxide retention. Creamy-yellow plaques on the eyelids are called xanthelasma and may indicate hyperlipidemia.

The information gained by the brief clinical examination of the eyes sometimes may indicate the true nature of oral diseases and necessity for additional investigation by ophthalmologist. Increased intercanthal distance is known as hypertelorism while decreased distance is called as hypotelorism.

Hypertelorism is seen in Down's syndrome, Cushing's syndrome, cretinism, Waardenburg syndrome, G syndrome, Aarskog syndrome, fracture of nasal bones and nasopharyngeal fibroma.

Altered interpupillary distance is due to diseases impairing development of brain.

Exophthalmos can be bilateral as in thyrotoxicosis or unilateral as in increased intraocular pressure. Enophthalmos can be seen in blowout fractures of the orbit.

Ptosis or drooping of one or both eyelids can be present congenitally, or in sclerosis, neoplastic/infectious diseases, tabes dorsalis and acute frontal sinusitis.

Periorbital edema can be observed in myxedema, fracture of inferior orbital margin, zygomatic arch fracture. Periorbital ecchymosis is observed in fractures of nasal bones, fracture of zygomatic arch.

Bitot's spots are plaque of yellowish sticky secretions seen in vitamin A deficiency.

Keratomalacia are the ulcerations, opacity, softening and destruction of cornea.

Interstitial keratitis is the grayish ground glass appearance of cornea.

Hyperthyroidism is characterized by exophthalmos, corneal ulcerations, infrequent blinking of eyes, widening of palpebral fissures.

Blue sclera can be a normal variant, or due to osteogenesis imperfecta, cherubism, fetal rickets, Marfan's syndrome, osteopetrosis. Brown sclera is observed in alkaptonuria. Argyll Robertson pupil is due to miosis associated with tabes dorsalis.

Some Oculo-oral syndromes of dental significance are:

- *Sjögrens' syndrome:* Dryness and stomatitis causing conjunctivitis, diminished secretions of mouth and pharynx.
- *Steven-Johnson syndrome:* Conjunctivitis associated with fever and stomatitis.
- *Behçet's syndrome:* Iritis, stomatitis, urethritis.

Nose

Appearance of external nasal pyramid has to be observed carefully. Nose can be:

- *Saddle shaped:* Syphilis (osteocartilaginous) or leprosy (cartilaginous)
- Humped
- Laterally deviated

Saddle shape deformity just seen above the tip of nose due to loss of support at dangerous area of the nose where it is supported by septal cartilage is known as boxer's nose.

Epistaxis results in Le Fort II and III fractures, malignancies and severe hypertension.

Nasal obstruction can be due to polyps, adenoids, septal deviations, tumors or large inflamed turbinate.

Relationship of mouth breathing to nasal breathing is of major concern to periodontal and orthodontic therapy. So, dental appliances for breaking the habit will not be of any value unless underlying cause is removed.

Extremities

The hands are usually exposed and easy to examine. They give important information on many conditions:

- Hypovolemic and cardiogenic shock may result in pale, cold and sweaty hands while distributive shock may result in warm, clammy hands.
- Nail changes can give information about systemic illness; a specific condition called clubbing may indicate serious cardiac or respiratory disease.
- Patients with arthritis can have specific bony deformities and nodules on the hands, sometimes associated with muscle wasting if severe.
- Liver disease can cause yellow discoloration, red palms (palmar erythema) and easy bruising. A flexion contraction of the 4th finger (Dupuytren's contracture) is associated with alcoholism, manual work or is familial.
- Pallor of the palmar crease may indicate anemia.
- Some patients have a tremor; this can be caused by cerebellar disease, movement disorders such as Parkinson's disease, carbon dioxide retention, anxiety or hyperthyroidism.
- An essential tremor is a benign condition where no medical cause is found.
- Cigarette smokers may have nicotine staining of their index and middle fingers. Some patients may wear medical alert bracelets.

Nails

Clubbing of finger nails is due to proliferation of vascular connective tissue underneath the nail beds as a result of chronic hypoxia/chronic toxemia. It is not expected that a dentist may be able to diagnose the diseases of finger nails in general. Sufficient knowledge of deviation from the normal and to relate changes in nails to systemic disorders of mouth is must. It is observed in:

- Infective endocarditis
- Coronary heart disease (CHD)
- Emphysema
- Lung abscess
- Bronchiectasis
- Crohn's disease
- Ulcerative colitis
- Myxedema.

Onychophagia (habit of eating nails) is associated with malocclusion, trauma to teeth and gingivitis. This may lead to small fractures of incisal edges of anterior teeth which reflects the psychological unrest of the patient.

Leukonychia (white nail) are due to trauma. Onycholysis is due to fungal infection. Beau's lines (Transverse Grooves) are seen in psoriasis and Darier's disease. Koilonychia is seen in Plummer-Vinson syndrome.

Skin

Thorough examination of skin, i.e. texture, color, eruptions, scars, etc. is of considerable importance because it frequently not only reflects manifestations of systemic diseases and health of individual but also because it may be of considerable importance in differential diagnosis of dermatologic lesions that appear in oral cavity or simultaneously on skin and oral cavity. Eruptions over the skin may be of characteristic distribution in different stages.

Koebner's phenomenon: Linear production of skin lesions by trauma in an uninvolved area of skin in the presence of other lesions nearby.

Zosteriform: Grouping of lesions in swaths.

Auspitz sign: Pin point bleeding spots seen after removing of overlying scale in psoriasis.

Nikolsky's sign: Involves superficial layers of skin which slip free from lower layers with slight rubbing pressure, with underlying areas appearing wet, moist and painful. Seen in Reiter's disease, toxic epidermal necrolysis (TEN) and pemphigus.

Color of skin of the patient has to be observed carefully. Underlying basis for alteration in the color of skin may be related to changes in the vascular bed, blood, bile pigments, metallic pigments and melanin. Thus, any physiological and pathological changes that may affect these various factors can give rise to alterations.

- Brown discoloration of the skin
  - Physiological variant
  - Melanin producing tumors
  - Addison's disease
  - Von Recklinghausen disease
  - Nutritional deficiency states: Pellagra
  - Hormonal imbalance: Chloasma gravidarum (Pregnancy)
  - Albright's disease
  - Neurofibromatosis
  - Cushing's disease
  - Peutz-jegher syndrome
- Pallor/Yellowish pigmentation
  - Hepatic disorders
  - Blockage of bile ducts
  - Renal failure
  - Anemia
  - Diabetes
  - Myxedema
  - Hypopituitarism
- Redness/Erythema
  - Fever
  - Burns

- Exposure to sunlight
- Telangiectasia
- Ulcerations
- Polycythemia vera
- Petechiae/Purpura
- Inflammatory conditions

Pallor is the clinical assessment for the amount of blood circulation in the body. It is assessed by pressing the nail bed with a light pressure till the nail bed becomes pale and then leaving it and seeing how fast the blood flows back to fill the area which was previously pressed. If the blood level is good then immediately it is filled.

It can also be done by examining the inner eyelids of the patient, the patient is asked to look up and his lower eyelids are pressed down by gentle pressure, if the blood circulation is good then the eyelid mucosa appears normal or if the circulation is less then it appears pale. It can also be assessed by looking at the oral cavity, where pale appearance of mucosa can be seen in patients who have less blood circulation. It can be also assessed on the tongue which shows loss of papilla, pale appearance on tongue, parched tongue and formation of cricoid webs in the tonsillar region in severely anemic patients.

Icterus is the yellowish appearance seen in patients who have high serum glutamic-oxaloacetic transaminase (SGOT) and serum glutamic-pyruvic transaminase (SGPT) levels. It suggests loss or decreased liver function hence no medicines which gets dissolved or act on liver can be given. Jaundice must be distinguished from yellow or green skin color resulting from carotenemia or quinacrine ingestion. Eating large quantities of green and yellow vegetables, tomatoes, or yellow corn may result in excess carotene intake. The resultant yellow skin color is differentiated from jaundice by the absence of yellow color in mucous membranes and sclerae, the normal urine color, and the accentuation of yellow-brown carotenoid pigment in the palms, soles, and nasolabial folds. Quinacrine, commonly used for treatment of giardiasis, may produce a yellow skin color, but the urine remains normal. Serum bilirubin levels are normal in patients with yellow skin caused by carotenemia or quinacrine.

5

Examination of Head and Neck Region

Introduction

Any abnormality in size, shape and symmetry of the head is to be examined, related to diagnosis and treatment of diseases with in province of dentist. Normal skull shape depends on sequential closure of sutures. Usually, at the age of 5, skull attains its adult size.

- Microcephaly (small head) is seen in craniostenosis, i.e. premature closure of cranial sutures.
- Dolichocephaly/Scaphocephaly presents with long narrow face due to early fusion of sagittal suture.
- Brachycephaly is the presence of a wide head due to early closure of coronal suture.
- Oxycephaly/Turricephaly is pointed/tower skull.
- Lack of closure of anterior fontanel persists as a soft spot as seen in cleidocranial dysostosis and progeria.
- Gradual asymmetric enlargement of head (Acorn shape head) can be seen in acromegaly and Paget's disease.

Gentle palpation is done to locate any small nodules, tender areas or swelling, presence of any of the lesions of psoriasis, lichen planus, lupus erythematosus.

Symmetry

A person will normally have clinically acceptable bilateral symmetry, that is to say that the hands, arms, legs, feet, trunk, face and head will be the same on each side of the body. Of course, there could be minor variations. Major variations will include atrophies/hypertrophies that are due to neurological/muscular disturbances. Tumors may be seen as asymmetrical growth.

Facial Profile

Examination of facial profile may reveal about position of the teeth and jaws. This is formed by connecting soft tissue glabella (G), subnasal (Sn) and soft tissue pogonion (Pg). Interpretation is done in the form of:

- *Concave (Class I):* Facial and dental has vertical maxillary excess or vertical maxillary deficiency.
- *Straight profile (Class II):* It means maxillary protrusion or vertical maxillary excess or mandibular retrusion.
- *Convex (Class III):* It means maxillary retrusion or vertical maxillary deficiency.

Andy Gump type and hapsburg jaw is the characteristic sign of malocclusion, malfunction, or maldevelopment.

Frog face deformity is characterized by widened bridge of nose, exophthalmos, bulging deformity of cheek bones.

When face is inspected, size and location of landmarks on each side are compared. Facial expressions may show evidence of organic diseases and express range of emotions. Paralysis of one side of face is observed in Bell's palsy, Ramsay Hunt syndrome, Melkersson Rosenthal syndrome, parotid tumors, etc. Asymmetries encountered are seen in association with alveolar abscess, functional and organic malpositioning of jaws, tumors, post-traumatic swellings or parotid gland disorders such as:

- *Mikulicz's syndrome:* There is involvement of parotid gland by systemic diseases like leukemia, lymphomas, sarcoidosis.
- *Sjögren syndrome:* One-third of patients suffer from diffuse firm painless swelling of parotid gland.

Facial Appearance in Different Diseases

- *Hyperthyroidism:* Exophthalmos, startled and anxious appearance.
- *Hypothyroidism:* Face appears puffy and swollen.
- *Down's syndrome:* Eyes slant upwards and outwards, nose appears broad and flat.
- *Parkinson's disease/Scleroderma/Muscular dystrophies:* Mask like expression less face.
- *Cushing's syndrome:* Round face, i.e. moon facies.
- *Thalassemia:* Mongoloid facies, frontal bossing, prominence of malar bones and pallor of skin due to anemia.
- *Leonine facies:* Leprosy and creeping periosteitis.
- *Adenoid facies:* Thin face and pinched nose, averted upper lips, receded chin, and expressionless face.
- *In dehydration:* Dry wrinkled skin with sunken cheeks and hollow eyes.

Temporomandibular Joint Examination

It is a ginglymoarthrodial joint capable of hinge type movements and gliding movements, with bony components enclosed and connected by a fibrous capsule. Mandibular condyle forms the lower part of the bony joint and glenoid fossa forms upper part of the joint. Space between condyle and fossa is occupied by collagenous fibrous tissue of variable thickness, called articular disc. Normal movement of the mandible depends on proper function of the temporomandibular joint (TMJ). Externally, the preauricular area lies directly over the joint.

Inspection

Begin by inspecting the preauricular area for swelling or erythema. The doctor should be in front of the patient and hold the patients head with both hands in such a way that his last finger is just inside the ear, the ring figure at the TMJ and the other fingers are at his forehead and above stabilizing the head to be straight. The patient should then be asked to open and close his mouth till he can feel the TMJ opening and closing normally. Following observations can be made:

- Gait of opening should be smooth, continuous and asynchronous
- Check for the opening of the mouth measuring distance between incisal edges of maxillary anterior teeth to incisal edges of mandibular anterior teeth. Maximum incisal opening in males is 40–50 mm and in females is 35–45 mm.
- Check for any deviation while opening the mouth. The mandible often deviates toward the affected side during opening because of muscle spasm or mechanical locking by a displaced meniscus. In closed position look for any deviation in midline. The maximum lateral deviation is 7–10 mm.
- Look for any obstruction during lateral and protrusive movements.
- Muscles of mastication and joint are observed carefully during joint movements.

Any condition (tumor, muscle spasm, fracture, ankylosis, displaced meniscus) that prevents the normal translation of one condyle will not prevent the contralateral condyle from sliding forward normally. The result is deviation of the chin toward the affected side. If translation of the condyles is prevented bilaterally, mandibular opening is restricted, usually to less than 25 mm.

Palpation

Palpate directly over the joint while the patient opens and closes the mandible, and the extent of mandibular condylar movement can be assessed. Normally, condylar movement is easily felt. Have the patient close slowly, and you will feel the condyle move posteriorly against your finger. Tenderness elicited by this maneuver is invariably associated with articular inflammation. Palpate the superficial temporal artery for nodularity and tenderness.

Muscles are palpated for the signs of tenderness, enlargement, spasm or tonicity. Bilateral palpation is the method of choice since movements of joints demand contralateral action of joints and muscles. Muscles responsible for mandibular movements are temporalis, masseter, medial and lateral pterygoid. Accessory muscles are sternocleidomastoid, trapezius, splenius capitis and digastrics. TMJ palpation can be done in 2 ways preauricular and lateral. TMJ should be palpated in immediate preauricular area by pressing gently over the lateral aspect of the joint. Little finger is placed in external auditory meatus and gentle forward pressure is applied. In this way, both lateral and posterior aspects of the joint can be palpated.

Muscles of Mastication

Masseter Muscle

It is inspected by asking the patient to clench his teeth and looking for the prominence of the muscle. Muscle is palpated bimanually by placing one finger intraorally and other on the cheek; extraorally muscle can be palpated by pressing the muscle against ramus of the mandible.

Temporalis

Origin can be palpated by asking the patient to clench his teeth. Digital palpation is preformed between superior and inferior temporal lines just above the ear, extending forward. Intraorally insertion can be palpated by running the finger up towards anterior border of ascending ramus where tendon inserts into coronoid process.

Lateral Pterygoid

It is best examined by recording its response to resisted functions/movements. Patient is asked to open his mouth in vertical direction and side-to-side movements against resistance, if there is a spasm of lateral pterygoid muscle tenderness will be reported in preauricular region. It is difficult to assess this muscle intraorally.

Medial Pterygoid

The muscle is palpated intraorally by placing the middle finger medially to pterygomandibular raphe and muscle is pressed laterally against inner surface of ramus of mandible.

Areas of identified muscle spasm or tenderness can be injected with local anesthesia, 2% lidocaine or 0.5% bupivacaine without epinephrine, or can be sprayed with fluoromethane or ethyl chloride to determine if these areas are the cause of the patient's symptoms.

Percussion

It can be either direct (by reflex action of mandible) or indirect (in the presence of cavities/fractures of bones.

Auscultation

This is done by placing the stethoscope at preauricular region. Use of stereo-stethoscope is better, as it has 2 diaphragms which can be placed on both the sides and sounds can be compared on both the sides, i.e. snapping, clicking, crepitus. The normal joint functions relatively quietly. Clicking is heard due to anterior disc displacement with reduction. Crepitus is occurrence of prolonged continuous noise in joint during movements and commonly seen in patients with degenerative joint diseases such as osteoarthrosis/acute inflammation.

Lock jaw is a condition with anterior disc displacement without reduction, where there is limited mouth opening.

Disorders of temporomandibular joint (TMJ) can be classified as:

- *Muscular:* Myofascial pain disorder syndrome (MPDS), masticatory muscle spasm, myositis.
- *Inflammatory:* Synovitis, rheumatoid arthritis, inflammatory arthritis, collagen vascular diseases.
- *Skeletal:* Osteoarthritis, disc displacement, disc degeneration, synovial adhesions, capsular fibrosis.
- Neoplastic
- *Congenital:* Condylar agenesis, hypoplasia, hypertrophy and hyperplasia, bifid condyle.
- *Traumatic injuries:* Intracapsular fractures, condylar neck fractures, dislocation, subluxation.

Examination of the Neck

Examination of the neck is a natural extension of a routine dental examination and includes the examination of the submandibular and cervical lymph nodes, midline structures, and presence of any swellings.

With the patient's neck extended note the clavicle and the sternocleidomastoid and trapezius muscle. Inspect the neck standing in front of the patient for any scars, or any swellings (either midline or lateral), color changes, dilation and pulsation of veins.

Palpation is done with examiner standing behind the patient. Palpate the hyoid bone, thyroid and cricoid cartilages, and trachea, noting any displacement or tenderness. If local or generalized thyroid enlargement is suspected, check to ascertain whether the mass moves when the patient swallows. Observe the external jugular vein as it crosses the sternocleidomastoid muscle, and with the patient at an angle of approximately 45° to the horizontal, note any distension or pulsation in the vein. Distension of >2 cm above the sternal notch is abnormal (right sided heart failure). Place the diaphragm of the stethoscope over the point of carotid pulse, and listen to the bruits or other disturbances of the rhythm that may indicate partial occlusion of the carotid artery.

Lymphadenopathy may be the only clinical finding or one of several nonspecific findings, and the discovery of swollen lymph nodes will often raise the suspicion of serious illness such as lymphoma, acquired immunodeficiency syndrome or metastatic cancer. The physician's task is to efficiently differentiate the few patients with serious illness from the many with self-limited disease. Most neck masses of specific cause occur in rather predictable location within typical age groups, which allows a systemic approach to develop a working diagnosis and differential diagnosis and management plan for a patient presenting with a neck mass. A wide range of diseases may present with lesions in the neck, but the most common complaint is of swelling and/or pain in the lymph node.

The various causes of lymphadenopathy are listed in **Table 1**.

The dental surgeon can often detect serious diseases through neck examination. Tenderness and swelling should be documented. Lymph nodes that are tender may be inflammatory (lymphadenitis). Lymph nodes swollen from acute infections are usually tender, soft and discrete, while chronic infections give firm lymph nodes. Nodes that are increasing in size and hard, or fixed to tissues may be malignant **(Table 2)**. Nodes that are enlarged and firm and matted or rubbery may be due to leukemia. In the lymphomas particularly, the nodes may be rubbery, matted together and fixed to deeper structures.

Table 1: Causes of lymphadenopathy

Infections	*Viral:* Infectious mononucleosis, Cytomegalovirus, HIV infection, Herpes simplex, Rubella, Measles, Adenovirus *Bacterial:* Syphilis, Tuberculosis, Brucellosis, Cat-scratch disease, Tularemia, *Streptococcus*, *Staphylococcus*, Diphtheria, Leprosy, Atypical mycobacterial infection *Fungal:* Histoplasmosis, Coccidioidomycosis *Parasitic:* Toxoplasmosis, Filariasis, Leishmaniasis **Chlamydial** **Rickettsial**
Malignant diseases	*Hematologic:* Hodgkin's, Non-Hodgkin's, Hairy cell leukoplakia, T-cell lymphoma, ALL, CLL, Malignant histiocytosis, Multiple myelosis with amyloidosis *Metastatic:* From primary sites
Immunologic diseases	Rheumatoid arthritis Systemic lupus erythematosus Sjögren's syndrome Primary biliary cirrhosis Drug hypersensitivity Mixed connective tissue disease Graft v/s Host disease Serum sickness
Lipid storage disease	Gaucher's disease, Niemann-Pick disease
Endocrine diseases	Adrenal insufficiency, Hyperthyroid, Thyroiditis
Medications	Allopurinol, Atenolol, Captopril, Carbamazepine, Hydralazine, Penicillin, Quinidine, Sulfonamides, Cephalosporins, Primidone, Pyrimethamine, Diphenylhydantoin, Gold, Sulindac
Others	Mucocutaneous lymph node syndrome (Kawasaki disease) Castleman's disease Sarcoidosis Histiocytosis X Lymphomatoid granulomatosis Kikuchi's disease Dermatopathic lymphadenitis

Source: Allhiser JN, Mcknight TA, Shank JC. Lymphadenopathy in a family practice. J Fam Pract. 1981;12:27-32.

Table 2: Various consistencies of lymph nodes in different conditions

Consistency	*Condition*
• Stony hard	• Carcinoma
• Soft/cystic	• Cold abcess
• Rubbery	• Hodgkins lymphoma
• Matted	• Tuberculosis
• Firm	• Syphilis

Source: Abba AA, Khalil MZ. Clinical approach to lymphadenopathy. Ann Nigerian Med. 2012;6:11-7.

In the systemic infective disorders the nodes are usually firm, discrete, tender and mobile.

The location of a lump or swelling in the neck will often give a good indication of the tissue of origin, and the age of the patient may help suggest the most likely diagnoses. The duration of the lesion is also relevant: one that has been present since an early age is likely to be of congenital origin, while a lump appearing in later life and persisting may be malignant.

- *Inspection:* It is done for number, position, size, surface of the skin, presence of any scar, sinus or ulcer. Skin over the swelling may show various features in different conditions such as:
  - *Acute lymphadenitis:* Redness, edema and Brawny induration.
  - *Chronic lymphadenitis:* Does not show such acuteness.
  - *Tuberculous lymphadenitis:* Usually cold till the skin becomes red and glossy and ready to burst.
  - *Lymphosarcoma:* Tense, shiny with dilated subcutaneous veins.
  - *Secondary carcinoma:* Fixed.
- *Palpation:* It is done to for number, situation, local temperature, fixity—to overlying skin or deeper structures, drainage area and consistency. Mobility should be checked in both horizontal and vertical plane. Malignancy shows fixity to the underlying skin. Discrete swellings in the neck may occasionally be caused by disorders in: salivary glands, thyroid gland and other structures. More diffuse swelling of the neck may be caused by: Infection, edema, malignant infiltration, surgical emphysema.

Neck nodes are better palpated while standing at the back of the patient. Neck is slightly flexed to achieve relaxation of the muscles. Palpate for lymph nodes in the neck, commencing with the most superior nodes and working down to the clavicle in the following order, so that none is missed:

1. Upper horizontal nodes
2. External jugular nodes
3. Internal jugular nodes
4. Spinal accessory nodes
5. Transverse cervical nodes
6. Anterior jugular nodes
7. Juxtavisceral nodes

Begin palpating by placing the flat surface of the fingertips at the same position on both sides of the patient's neck and palpate the parotid region by rolling the fingers against the maxilla, infront of the ear. The patient's head is moved from side-to-side sufficiently to allow free access to the structures beneath the area. Then start palpating bilaterally down the angles of the jaws, along the bases of the mandible and below the mandible to the midline. In the midline, tissues and nodes in the submental region are palpated by pressing them upwards against the symphysis of the jaw. Submandibular nodes can be palpated by rolling the fingers against the inner surface of the mandible with patients' neck tilted. Palpate at the mastoid and base of the skull for posterior auricular and occipital nodes.

The superficial cervical nodes lie above the sternomastoid muscle; the deep cervical nodes lie between the sternomastoid muscle and cervical fascia. To examine the latter, ask the patient to sit erect and to turn his or her head to one side to relax the sternomastoid; use thumb and fingers to palpate under the anterior and posterior borders of the relaxed muscle, and repeat the procedure on the opposite side. Next, palpate the posterior cervical nodes in the posterior triangle close to the anterior border of the trapezius muscle. Finally, check for supraclavicular nodes just above the clavicle, lateral to the attachment of the sternomastoid muscle. Few important and common swellings are listed in **Table 3**.

Generalized lymph node enlargement, including cervical nodes occurs in:

- Systemic infections, such as the glandular fever syndromes caused by Epstein-Barr virus, cytomegalovirus or toxoplasmosis and HIV/AIDS. Lymphadenitis in tuberculosis may lead to neck swelling (scrofula) and suppuration (cold abscess).
- Idiopathic lesions such as sarcoidosis and mucocutaneous lymph node syndrome (Kawasaki disease), these are not known to be infective.
- Neoplasms of the lymphoreticular system, such as lymphomas and leukemias, usually cause enlargement of many or all cervical lymph nodes and in some there is clinical involvement of the whole reticuloendothelial

Table 3: Few important and common midline swellings, lateral swellings and swellings that move on deglutition

Midline swellings	*Lateral swellings*	*Swellings that move on deglutition*
• Enlarged submental lymph nodes • Ludwig's angina • Thyroglossal cyst • Sublingual dermoid cyst • Goiter of thyroid isthmus	• Branchial cyst • Laryngocele • Enlarged submandibular gland • Deep/plunging ranula • Carotid body tumor • Cystic hygroma • Lipoma	• Thyroid swelling • Thyroglossal cyst (moves up with protrusion of tongue) • Laryngocele

Source: McPhee SJ, Papadakis MA, Tierney LM. 2007 Current Medical Diagnosis and Treatment. New York, NY: McGraw Hill; 2006.

system, which is generalized lymph node enlargement (detectable clinically in the neck, groin and axilla) and enlargement of both liver and spleen (hepatosplenomegaly).

Intraoral Examination

After the general appraisal of the patient the examiner may continue with detailed examination of the mouth, using all the necessary principles of physical examination. Good illumination is a prerequisite for a thorough examination of the mouth. The patient should be seated comfortably for proper instrumentation and access to all areas of the mouth.

Lips

Inspection of the lips is performed first as these are the first to attract attention in approaching the mouth. Inspection is directed towards changes in color, form, texture and obvious lesions. Normally, the lips are smooth and pink in color, and in younger persons fissuring is minimal. With advancing age a curl develops in the corner of the mouth, the labiomarginal sulcus. Patient is asked to open his lips slightly and line represented by lower edge of upper lip is noted for its relationship to teeth, which can vary in position from incisal edges to cervical third of maxillary teeth.

Any disease that affects the number of RBC, amount of reduced hemoglobin, or the oxygen carrying capacity of blood may lead to various color changes of lips. A bluish tint may be observed in cardiac failure, chronic obstructive pulmonary disease (COPD) and high altitude; in congenital shunts color are almost purple; varying degrees of blue color of cyanosis may be seen in emphysema. Lips become thickened, desquamated, and bluish purple in color due to prolonged exposure to sun and various elements. In mouth breathers lower lips become dry and chapped. Bell's Palsy can be tested by asking the patient to smile and noticing the deviation of the mouth to unaffected side, and also the inability of the patient to whistle.

Common lip lesions important from the examination point of view are as under:

- *Developmental anomalies:*
  - Lip pits/Commissural pits
  - *Double lip:* When the lips are tensed or pursed an additional fold of soft tissue is felt just inside the lip.
  - Cheilitis granulomatosa
  - Cheilitis glandularis
- *White lesions:* Perleche, Lichen planus, Actinic keratosis, Cigarette smoker's lip, Squamous cell carcinoma, Focal epithelial hyperplasia.
- *Ulcerative lesions:* Traumatic ulcer, Aphthous ulcer, Herpes labialis, Erythema multiforme, Keratoacanthoma.
- Mucocele, Hemangioma, Contact allergy.
- Some common syndromes associated with lip anomalies are:
  - *Ascher's syndrome:* It is characterized by the presence of double lip, blepharosclerosis and thyroid enlargement.

  - *Van der Woude syndrome:* The clinical features include presence of lip pits and cleft palate.
  - *Melkersson-Rosenthal syndrome:* Diagnostic features of the syndrome include cheilitis granulomatosa, facial paralysis and scrotal tongue.
- Other lesions may be
  - Angular cheilitis
  - Presence of ectopic sebaceous glands is commonly found at vermillion border of upper lip
  - Swollen lips due to trauma, angioneurotic edema
  - Thickened lips observed in cretinism, acromegaly and hyperpituitarism.

Tongue

Tongue is a muscular organ associated with the function of deglutition, taste and speech. It acts as an easily accessible organ for the assessment of health of an individual and shows the state of hydration of the body. It is said that tongue is the mirror of the gastrointestinal system and any abnormal functioning of the stomach and intestines will be reflected on the tongue. Some characteristic changes occur in the tongue in some particular diseases. That is why the examination of the tongue is very essential and will give some clues for diagnosis. All doctors examine the tongue and they consider the changes in size, shape, color, moisture, coating, nature of papillae and movements, etc.

Examination of tongue is done first in the normal resting position to look for its association with the incisal/occlusal edges of the teeth. Normally, the tongue rests behind the lower anteriors and approximates occlusal surface of posterior teeth. Then a gauze piece is wrapped around the tip of the tongue and the tongue is gently pulled outside to observe the dorsum of the tongue and tongue is guided in either direction to look for the lateral borders of the tongue. Other examination techniques include:

- Cine radiographic studies of oral cavity and pharynx during drinking, chewing, suckling, phonation, etc.
- Computer assisted tomography
- Pulsed and real time ultrasound
- Isotopic scanning technique
- Electromyography
- Scanning electron microscopy
- Transmission electron micrograph (TEM)

Changes in the movements of the tongue may be observed in the following:

1. In one sided paralysis of the body (hemiplegia) tongue moves towards the paralyzed side on protrusion.
2. Tremulus movement of the tongue is seen in diseases like thyrotoxicosis, delirium tremens and Parkinsonism. Tremor is also seen in nervous patients.
3. In progressive bulbar palsy there will be wasting and paralysis of the tongue with fibrillation. Eventually the tongue gets shrivelled and lies functionless in the floor of the mouth. This condition is associated with drooling of saliva and speech impairment.

4. In chorea (involuntary rhythmic movements) the patient may not be able to keep the protruded tongue in rest, it will be moving involuntarily.

The moistness of the tongue gives some indication about the state of hydration of the body. Water volume depletion leads to peripheral circulatory failure characterized by weakness, thirst, restlessness, anorexia, nausea, vomiting, dry and parched tongue. Dryness of the tongue is seen in diarrhea, later stages of severe illness, advanced uremia, hypovolemic shock, heat exhaustion, hyponatremia, acute intestinal obstruction, starvation and prolonged fasting.

Change in color of tongue can be observed in the following:

1. Central cyanosis
2. Jaundice
3. *Advanced uremia:* The tongue becomes brown in color.
4. *Ketoacidosis:* Seen mainly in diabetes mellitus. The tongue becomes brown with a typical ketone smell from the mouth.
5. *Riboflavin deficiency:* Deficiency of vitamin B_2 produces megenta color of the tongue with soreness and fissures of lips. In mild states glossitis with soreness at tip and lateral margins alongwith atrophy of filiform papillae is seen and the tongue appears red and granular. In severe cases tongue becomes glazed and smooth giving a magenta color.
6. *Niacin deficiency:* Deficiency of vitamin B_3 and some other B complex vitamins results in bright scarlet or beefy red tongue with small shallow ulcers. It is also known as Hunter's glossitis/Moeller's glossitis.
7. *Anemia:* In severe anemia tongue becomes pale.

Papillae are small projections on the tongue associated with taste. There are different types of papillae on the healthy tongue. In the following diseases some abnormal changes are noted in these papillae:

1. *Hairy tongue:* This condition is due to elongation of filiform papillae seen in poor oral hygiene, general debility and indigestion.
2. *Geographic tongue:* Multiple annular areas of desquamation of papillae appear on the tongue which shifts from area to area in few days.
3. Median rhomboid glossitis.
4. *Nutritional deficiency:* In nutritional deficiency there is glossitis (inflammation of tongue) leading to papillary hypertrophy followed by atrophy. In nutritional megaloblastic anemia the tongue becomes smooth.
5. *Thiamine and riboflavin deficiency:* Deficiency of these vitamins causes hypertrophy of filiform and fungiform papillae.
6. *Niacin and iron deficiency:* In this condition there is atrophy of papillae. Smooth tongue is encountered in iron deficiency.
7. *Folic acid deficiency:* Swelling and redness of the tip and lateral border of the tongue, loss of filiform and fungi form papillae, silky, smooth and fiery red tongue is observed.
8. *Vitamin A deficiency:* Furrowed tongue is observed in this condition.
9. Cyanocobalamin deficiency.
10. *Scarlet fever:* In this streptococcal infection there are bright red papillae standing out of a thick white fur. Later the white coat disappear leaving enlarged papillae on the bright red surface and is called strawberry tongue.

Anomalies of the Tongue

- Developmental disorders
  - *Microglossia:* Uncommon developmental anomaly, most of the cases are reported with one group of overlapping conditions, i.e. Oromandibular-limb hypogenesis syndrome associated with hypodactylia, hypomelia, cleft palate, hypoplasia of the mandible.
  - *Macroglossia:* It may be of two types:
    i. Symmetrical as seen in Down's syndrome, acromegaly, myxedema, Sturge-Weber syndrome, Hurler's syndrome and amyloidosis.
    ii. Asymmetrical as seen in hemangioma, lymphangioma, neurofibromatosis, angioedema and hemifacial hypertrophy.

    Macroglossia is also found to be associated with Beckwith-Wiedemann syndrome.
  - *Ankyloglossia (Tongue tie):* It results due to abnormally thick and short lingual frenum. In rare cases there may be complete absence of lingual frenum.
  - Long narrow extensible tongue is seen in Ehlers-Danlos syndrome and Tuberous-sclerosis.
  - *Median rhomboid glossitis:* It is a developmental and congenital defect due to persistence of tuberculum impair over the dorsum of the tongue. It is rhomboid or oval shaped area seen over the dorsum in midline just anterior to circumvallate papillae. It may appear as red, sharply demarcated depressed area on the dorsum of the tongue or raised tumor like mass with wide base and is firm pebbled smooth and pink in color.
  - *Geographic tongue/Benign migratory glossitis/Wandering rash/Areata migrans:* It appears as irregular, circinate, nonindurated, atrophic areas on the tongue that gradually widen, change shape and migrate over tongue. These lesions look like a geographic map. It is bordered by slightly elevated, distinct rim that varies from gray to white to light yellow.
  - *Fissured tongue/Scrotal tongue:* It is characterized by grooves that vary in depth and are noted along the dorsal and lateral aspects of the tongue.
  - *Cleft tongue:* Distinct clefts of the tongue are rare and are usually restricted to the tip of tongue. These are the true clefts rather than true fissures.
  - *Black hairy tongue (Lingua nigra):* It should not be confused with oral hairy leukoplakia which is usually manifested by the presence of hyperkeratotic vertical striations seen over the lateral border of the tongue.
  - *Lingual thyroid:* It is seen as a small nodule present near the root of the tongue, it can vary in size from a small nodule to big masses which can obstruct the airway.
  - *Lingual varicosities:* These are the abnormally dilated torturous veins seen over the ventral surface of the tongue, most commonly in elderly people.

- *Coated tongue:* Initially thought to be the symptom of GIT disturbances, now it is seen to be associated with poor oral hygiene, inadequate eating habits and altered mobility of tongue.
- Papillitis is the inflammation of lingual papillae.
- Depapillation/Atrophy of papillae is seen in trauma (thermal, chemical or mechanical) and deficiency states.
- *Pigmentation:* Melanotic pigmentation, pallor, exogenous pigmentation of filiform papillae, tattooing of lateral margins of tongue, extravasation of red blood cells around lingual varicosities.
- Mucous patch of syphilis.
- *Ulcerations of the tongue:* These can be further divided as
  - *Acute ulcers:* These result due to sudden trauma to the tongue due to epileptic seizures, blow to jaw, foreign body impingement and dental equipment.
  - *Chronic ulcers:* These are caused by uncontrolled grinding of the teeth or rough surfaces of the restoration or jagged tooth surfaces.
  - Shallow persistent ulcers are present in nutritional deficiencies, hematological problems, xerostomia, aphthous ulcers, Behçets syndrome and pemphigus.
  - Deep ulcers are observed in chronic granulomatous infections like tuberculosis, sarcoidosis, geotrichosis, mucormycosis, etc.
  - Cancerous ulcers are having everted edges with hard base.
  - *Syphilitic ulcers:* Syphilitic fissures are longitudinal in direction. In primary syphilis extragenital chancre is seen on the tongue. In secondary syphilis multiple shallow ulcers are seen on the under surface and sides of the tongue. In tertiary syphilis gumma may be seen on the midline of the dorsum of the tongue.
- Fibroma of tongue is seen due to trauma.
- Glossodynia/Glossopyrosis seen in deficiency states.

Labial and Buccal Mucosa

Inspection begins with reflection of upper and lower lips and inspection of color and texture of labial mucosa. Palpation can be bidigital as well as bilateral. Look for any color changes on labial mucosa. Labial mucosa shows varying degrees of nodularity associated with numerous mucous glands. Several folds of tissue, called frena traverse the vestibular fornix. The cheek is reflected and buccal mucosa is inspected for color, texture, and lesions. Color can vary from pink to bluish-gray **(Table 4)**. Labial and buccal mucosa may show petechial hemorrhages and ecchymoses of purpura and leukemia. Trauma may cause ulcerations, fibromas and mucus retention cysts. Certain conditions termed as normal variants may be observed, which are normal but appear as pathology such as:

- *Linea alba buccalis:* It is defined as thin, white line at the occlusal level, accentuated by trauma.
- Buccal pad of fat is observed in front of anterior border of masseter as rounded eminence containing fat tissue.

Table 4: Alteration in color of the labial and buccal mucosa

White lesions	Leukoedema, lichen planus, verrucous carcinoma, white spongy nevus, traumatic keratosis, candidiasis, psoriasis, oral submucous fibrosis, radiation mucositis, uremic stomatitis
Red and white lesions	Chronic mechanical trauma, erosive lichen planus, speckled leukoplakia, hypertrophic or hyperplastic candidiasis, lupus erythematosus, chemical or thermal burn, allergic or radiation mucositis, mucous patch, pemphigoid, erythema-multiforma
Brownish pigmentation	Physiological melanin deposition, Peutz-jegher's syndrome, Café-au-lait spots, Addison's disease, Cushing's disease, acromegaly, hypothyroidism, liver cirrhosis, chronic kidney insufficiency
Pallor	Anemia
Yellowish discoloration	Jaundice

Source: Regezi JA, Sciubba JJ, Pogrel MA. Atlas of Oral and Maxillofacial Pathology. Philadelphia, Pa: WB Saunders;1999.

- *Parotid papillae:* It is soft in consistency located opposite to 2nd molar, when palpated; and if parotid gland is manipulated, a quantity of serous fluid may be expressed.
- Retromolar papillae bis located behind distal molars, there are soft tissue eminences.
- Fordyce granules are characterized by heterotrophic collections of sebaceous glands at various sites in the oral cavity.

Palate

The mucus membrane of hard palate is firmly attached to underlying bone and presents some degree of keratinization; the factors give it a pale pink color often with a bluish gray hue. Palate is to be examined for the presence of any cysts, tori, clefts/perforations and inflammatory hyperplasias. Color changes in the palate may be due to:

- *Inflammation from traumatic agents:* Erythematous in color.
- *Denture wearers:* Bluish white to brilliant red in color (Denture stomatitis).
- *Smoker's patch:* A brown staining of keratinized surface may occur especially in that area in which a pipe stem or cigar rests.
- *Smoker's palate:* Extensive keratinization of the palate with involvement of orifices of the mucous glands, diffuse silver-white color with punctate red areas (Stomatitis nicotina palati).
- *Blood dyscrasias:* Pallor, ecchymoses, petechiae.

Also check the movements of the soft palate and uvula when the patient is asked to say "ah". Absence of palatal reflex is seen in hysteria and paralysis of palate.

Floor of the Mouth

Examination of floor of mouth can be best accomplished by inspection and palpation. The former is carried out by having the patient elevate his tongue while the examiner retracts the tissue from the mandible with a mouth mirror. Structures occupying the floor of the mouth are:

- Sublingual glands and ducts
- Superior part of submaxillary glands and ducts
- Lymph nodes along the inferior border of mandible
- Lingual nerves and branches.

Sublingual sulcus is traversed in midline by lingual frenum and on each side of it lays a small round nodule called sublingual caruncle which contains openings of submaxillary and sublingual gland ducts.

Changes in the color of the floor may be present with inflammatory changes, hyperkeratotic changes or due to associated systemic diseases. Look for presence of ulcerations as seen due to trauma or associated with primary or secondary herpes.

Palpation of floor of the mouth is best done bimanually with examiner facing the patient and the patient in an upright position with head and jaw turned slightly downward to get maximum relaxation of the muscles of the floor of the mouth. It begins in the midline and traverses the soft issue posteriorly without causing undue discomfort to the patient. At the same time lingual sulcus of mandible is palpated for exostosis, areas of tenderness, and loss of firmness.

A swelling in the floor of mouth should be palpated to determine its consistency and extent. Soft fluctuant masses are cystic in nature, and hard board like manifestations may be associated with cellulitis of sublingual space; hard firmly attached enlargement associated with the sublingual glands may be inflammatory or neoplastic. Bimanual palpation is done to determine the presence of stones in Wharton's duct along with occlusal radiographs.

Oropharynx

Normal color of this region appears to be moist bright pink with dilated veins and nodular prominences. Tonsils may vary greatly in size being large in children and projecting toward the midline of tonsillar fossa. Size and form of oropharynx vary considerably and are often related to the character of facies. Broad faced child has a broad enlarged oropharynx, whereas narrow faced child has a narrow and small oropharynx. Tongue depressor is used to visualize tonsillar area and oropharynx.

In the plane with the soft palate and on posterior wall of the pharynx is the ridge of tissues called Passavant's bar that closes the nasal cavity during deglutition. Waldeyer's ring is a band of lymphoid tissue that surrounds the pharynx.

Chief characteristics of chronically infected tonsils are persistent redness of the tonsil and adjacent mucosa with repeated attacks of tonsillitis and presence of lymphadenopathy of lymph nodes draining the tonsils. Enlarged tonsils may be associated with the habit of mouth breathing. Such enlargement of the tonsils may close the nasopharynx resulting in development of acquired swallowing reflex in the children. As a result of this the mandible and tongue move forward, leading to the development of tongue thrusting habit, which predisposes to malocclusion.

Gingiva

It is a band of soft tissue that surrounds the tooth in a collar like fashion with scalloped margins. Gingiva is divided into 3 parts: marginal gingiva, attached gingiva, and alveolar mucosa. Marginal gingiva is separated by attached gingiva by a free marginal groove; while attached gingiva is separated from alveolar mucosa by mucogingival junction.

Marginal gingiva consists of the free gingiva and gingival sulcus.

Free gingiva: The area of gingiva above the attachment at CEJ is called as free gingiva because it is not attached to any underlying tissue.

Gingival sulcus: It is an area extending from the margin to the attachment level of the gingiva. The gingiva is attached at the cemetoenamel junction (CEJ). The groove formed on the inner side of the gingiva (towards the tooth) between the gingival margin and the CEJ attachment is called gingival sulcus. For anterior teeth the gingival sulcus is normally 2–3 mm clinically above the CEJ. This can be assessed by passing the probe along the gingival sulcus. Histologically the gingival sulcus is 1.5–1.8 mm.

Attached gingiva is the gingiva seen below the gingival sulcus and it is attached to the underlying tissue (periosteal bone). For anterior teeth it is 3.5–4.5 mm in the maxilla and 3.3–3.9 mm in the mandible. In the posterior teeth the attached gingiva is 1.9 mm in maxilla and 1.8 mm in mandible.

Interdental gingiva is the gingiva present between the two teeth. In the anterior teeth the inter dental free gingiva is cone shaped while in the posterior teeth it is dome shaped and covers till the contact point of any two adjacent teeth.

Mucogingival junction: It is the junction where the attached gingiva joins with the mucosa of the oral cavity. It can be seen by retracting the lower or upper lip and seeing the movement of the mucosa just below the attached gingiva.

Careful visual inspection should be done to observe:
- Changes in color which depends upon changes in the vascular bed
- Presence or absence of keratinization
- Presence of reduced hemoglobin
- Presence of pigmentation
- Thickness of epithelium
- Interdental papillary contour and texture
- Marginal gingiva.

The consistency and texture can be evaluated by means of palpation.

The color of the attached and marginal gingiva is generally described as coral pink. The color varies among different persons and appears to be correlated with the cutaneous pigmentation. It is lighter in individuals with fair complexion than in dark-haired and black individuals. The alveolar mucosa is red, smooth and shiny rather pink and stippled. Color changes in the gingiva may be observed due to one of the following causes:

- Physiological pigmentation is due to presence of melanin. It may be increased to brownish pigmentation seen in Addison's disease, Peutz-Jegher's syndrome, Albright's disease and von-Recklinghausen disease.
- Metallic pigmentation due to lead (Burtonian line), Ag, Sn, Hg (linear black pigmentation) and amalgam tattoos.
- *Inflammatory conditions:* Acute gingivitis [Acute necrotizing ulcerative gingivitis (ANUG), herpetic gingivostomatitis], chronic gingivitis.
- *Systemic conditions:* Anemia, polycythemia, leukemia, jaundice, diabetes.
- *Tobacco use:* Hyperkeratotic grayish areas are seen.
- Local irritants.
- Accretions, films, plaque, necrotic tissue also can alter the color of the gingiva.

Color changes are frequently accompanied by textural changes. Normally, the gingiva gives stippled, orange peel appearance. The attached gingiva is stippled; the marginal gingiva is not. It is a feature of healthy gingiva and reduction or loss of stippling is a common sign of gingival disease. Loss of stippling is seen in early gingival disease, smooth texture is due to atrophy of epithelium, desquamation of superficial layers, stretching of epithelium from under lying edema/scar tissue. Surface texture is associated with hyperkeratosis. Friability, ulceration, and induration are important features of hyperkeratosis to be evaluated by inspection and palpation.

Changes in consistency: Normally, gingiva is firm and resilient in consistency, with the exception of movable free gingiva due to collagenous nature of underlying lamina propria. That means the gingiva cannot be lifted up as it is attached to the bone and has sufficient elasticity to take up stresses of occlusion. In people who do not have healthy gingiva, the gingiva appears swollen and the gingival margins become thickened.

Palpation with a slight pressure may be utilized to discover edema, pitting, fluctuance, induration and friability of tissues. Edema is seen in chronic inflammation. Fluctuance is seen in periodontal/gingival abscess, bullae/vesicle. Changes in contour: The contour or shape of the gingiva varies considerably and depends on the shape of the teeth and their alignment in the arch, the location and size of the area of proximal contact, and the dimensions of the facial and lingual gingival embrasures. Changes in contour are seen due to local or systemic changes in the gingiva, alteration in the form of teeth due to decay, traumatic occlusion, gingival hyperplasia, chronic irritation, mixed dentition period, improper tooth brushing/orthodontic tooth movements.

Level of epithelial attachment: Normally the level of epithelial attachment lies over the enamel or cementoenamel junction. Check for any alteration in level of attachment.

Depth of gingival sulcus: Normal depth is less than 3 mm. Look for gingival bleeding on probing the sulcus which is one of the indicative signs of gingival disease.

Acute necrotizing ulcerative gingivitis (ANUG) and chronic periodontitis show loss of interdental papillae. Gingival enlargement can be inflammatory and fibrotic.

Gingival recession is the exposure of tooth by the apical migration of gingiva. It may be physiological (associated with age) or pathological. It results due to faulty tooth brushing habits, tooth malposition, friction from soft tissues, gingival inflammation, abnormal frenum attachment and iatrogenic dentistry. Exposed root surfaces are susceptible to caries and also lead to hyperemia of the pulp and development of associated symptoms. Interproximal recession creates oral hygiene problems and resulting plaque accumulation. Abrasion or erosion of the cementum due to recession leaves an underlying dentinal surface that can be sensitive.

Sullivan and Atkins classified gingival recession into four morphologic categories:

1. Shallow-narrow
2. Shallow-wide
3. Deep-narrow
4. Deep-wide.

Classification according to Miller:

Class I: Marginal tissue recession does not extend to the mucogingival junction. There is no loss of bone or soft tissue in the interdental area. It can be narrow or wide.

Class II: Marginal tissue recession extends to or beyond the mucogingival junction. There is no loss of bone or soft tissue in the interdental area. It can be narrow or wide.

Class III: Marginal tissue recession extends to or beyond the mucogingival junction. There is loss of bone or soft tissue in the interdental area or malpositioning of the tooth.

Class IV: Marginal tissue recession extends to or beyond the mucogingival junction. There is severe bone and soft tissue loss interdentally or severe malpositioning of the tooth.

Hard Tissue Examination

It is done by using mouth mirror and explorer. Careful visual inspection should be done with an unaided eye and with mouth mirror under bright artificial light. Mouth mirror is used for retraction of the buccal mucosa and indirect illumination while the explorer is used to walk it along the grooves and ridges and to find any dipping of its pit or for a catch. Percussion is done with end of handle of mouth mirror. The following should be taken into consideration while examining the teeth:

- Number
- Size/Form/Shape
- Colors/Stains
- Carious lesions
- Occlusion
- Attrition/Erosion/Abrasion
- Fractures
- Vitality test.

Abnormalities of teeth can be grouped under two broad categories:

1. Developmental
2. Environmental

Developmental anomalies of teeth may be related to size, shape, number, structure and growth (eruption) of teeth.

On the basis of size, teeth can be either of the following:

- *Microdontia:* These are teeth of small size. They can be either true generalized, relative generalized or microdontia involving a single tooth. One of the common forms of localized microdontia is peg laterals that affect the maxillary lateral incisors.
- *Macrodontia:* These are teeth of size larger than normal. They can be either true generalized, relative generalized or microdontia involving a single tooth. A variant of the localized macrodontia is the type occasionally seen in hemihypertrophy of the face, where the teeth of the involved side may be considerably larger than the unaffected side.

The role hereditary factors in relative microdontia and macrodontia must be considered.

On the basis of number, teeth can be either of the following:

- *Hyperdontia:* Presence of more than usual number of teeth. It is the presence of supernumerary teeth. Relative conditions associated with hyperdontia are: Apert's syndrome, Cleidocranial dysplasia, Gardner's syndrome, etc.
- *Anodontia:* True anodontia or congenital absence of teeth, may be of 2 types, total and partial. Total anodontia, where all the teeth are missing may involve either of the dentition. It is a rare condition and is frequently associated with hereditary ectodermal dysplasia.

Hypodontia or oligodontia (true partial anodontia) is less than usual number of teeth. A familial tendency for this defect is present in many instances. Conditions associated with hypodontia are: Down's syndrome, Ectodermal dysplasia, Crouzon's disease, Ehler-Danlos syndrome, Focal dermal hypoplasia, Turner's syndrome, Palmoplantar keratosis, Cleft lip/palate among others.

On the basis of shape, teeth can be either of the following:

- *Gemination:* It is present when a developing tooth bud tends to divide by an invagination, which leads to incomplete formation of two teeth.

- *Fusion:* It is the union of two normally separated tooth germs. Depending on the stage of development of teeth at the time of the union, it may be complete or incomplete. It may also occur between a normal and a supernumerary tooth.
- *Concrescence:* It is a form of fusion which occurs after root formation. Teeth are united by cementum only.
- *Dilaceration:* This refers to an angulation or a sharp bend or curve, in the root or crown of a formed tooth.
- *Talon's cusp (Rubinstein-Taybi syndrome):* It is an anomalous structure resembling an eagle's talon, and projects lingually from the cingulum areas of a maxillary or mandibular permanent incisor.
- *Dens invaginatus (Dens in dente):* This developmental variation is thought to arise as a result of an invagination in the surface of crown of the tooth before calcification has occurred.
- *Dens evaginatus (Leong's premolar):* It occurs as an accessory cusp or a globule of enamel on the occlusal surface between the buccal and lingual cusps of premolars, either unilaterally or bilaterally.
- *Taurodontism:* Anomaly where there is enlargement of the body and pulp chamber of multirooted teeth at the expense of roots, with apical displacement of pulpal floor and bifurcation of the roots. Shaw classified them into: hypotaurodont, mesotaurodont and hypertaurodont.

  Syndromes associated with taurodontism are cranioectodermal dysplasia, Klinefelter's disease, Down's syndrome, microcephalic dwarfism, trichoonychodental disorders among others.
- *Supernumerary roots:* It is common and may involve any tooth.

On the basis of structure, teeth can be either of the following:

- *Amelogenesis imperfecta:* Group of the conditions that demonstrates alteration in the structure of enamel in the absence of systemic diseases. It may be differentiated into three basic types:
  1. *Hypoplastic:* Localized hypoplastic teeth show horizontal rows of pits, a linear depression in middle third of buccal surfaces and their color may vary from opaque white to translucent brown. Whereas, generalized hypoplastic teeth show pin-point to pin-head size pits across the surface of teeth.
  2. *Hypomaturative:* These teeth show mottled, opaque, brown-yellow discoloration. Enamel is softer than normal, tends to chip off and can be pierced with dental explorer. Snow-capped pattern is seen radiographically.
  3. *Hypocalcified:* Enamel is very soft, yellowish-brown-black in color.
- *Dentinogenesis imperfecta:* It is an autosomal dominant developmental disturbance of dentin in the absence of any systemic disorders. Color varies from gray to blue-brownish discoloration with distinct translucency/ opalescent hue. It is of two types:
  1. Dentinogenesis imperfecta 1
  2. Dentinogenesis imperfecta 2

- *Dentin dysplasia:* It is a rare disturbance of dentin formation characterized by normal enamel but atypical dentin formation with abnormal pulpal morphology. It is of 2 types radicular (type I) and coronal (type II). In coronal type color varies from blue to amber to brown translucency.
- *Regional odontodysplasia:* It is a developmental anomaly with extensive adverse effects on enamel, dentin and pulp. Erupted teeth demonstrate small, irregular crowns that are yellow to brown, often with a rough surface. They show a marked reduction in radiodensity on radiographs and assume a ghost appearance.

Disturbances in growth can result in the following:

- *Premature eruption:* A decidous tooth that has erupted into the oral cavity and is occasionally seen in infants.
- *Eruption sequestrum:* It is a tiny irregular spicule of bone overlying the crown of an erupting permanent molar, just prior to immediately following the eruption of the cusp tips.
- *Delayed eruption*
- *Multiple unerupted teeth:* Uncommon condition where there is more or less permanently delayed eruption of teeth.
- *Embedded or impacted teeth:* These teeth fail to erupt usually due to lack of eruptive force.
- *Submerged teeth (ankylosed deciduous teeth):* These deciduous teeth, mostly the mandibular second molars, have undergone a variable degree of root resorption and then have become ankylosed to the bone.

Environmental anomalies of teeth are:

- *Enamel hypoplasia:* It is a defect that occurs as a result of any disturbance in enamel matrix proteins, occurring in the form of grooves, pits or large areas of missing enamel. Factors associated with enamel hypoplasia are:
  - Birth related trauma
  - Chemicals, i.e. Antineoplastics, fluorides, tetracycline, thalidomide, vitamin D
  - Chromosomal abnormality such as trisomy 21
  - Malnutrition
  - *Metabolic disorders:* Cardiac/celiac/hepatobiliary/hyperbilirubinemia, etc.
  - Neurological.
- *Turner's hypoplasia:* It is due to extension of infection from the deciduous tooth to the developing tooth bud. Altered tooth is called as Turners' tooth, which appears as focal areas of white, yellow, or brown discoloration involving entire crown of tooth.
- *Dental fluorosis:* It results due to the ingestion of excessive amount of fluoride, which results in retention of amelogenin proteins leading to hypomineralized enamel. It may be:
  - *Mild:* Chalky white flecks or spotted enamel.
  - *Moderate:* White opaque areas involving more of tooth surface.
  - *Severe:* Pitting and brownish staining.
- *Syphilitic hypoplasia:* Congenital syphilis is characterized by the presence of Hutchinson's incisors (screw-driver shaped) and mulberry molars (occlusal surface resembles mulberry).

Tooth Wear

- Attrition is the physiological loss of tooth structure caused by tooth to tooth contact during occlusion and mastication. Clinically, polished, flat, smooth, wear-facets are seen over cusp tips or ridges with flattening of incisal edges.
- Abrasion is the pathological loss of tooth structure secondary to the action of external agents, like tooth-brushing, abrasive toothpastes, bobby pins, pipe stems, etc. Clinically, V-shaped or wedge shaped ditch is seen on root side of cementoenamel junction (CEJ), in teeth with some gingival recession.
- Erosion is the loss of tooth substance by chemical process that does not involve known bacterial action. Clinically, polished, smooth, scooped out depressions are seen on the enamel surface adjacent to CEJ.
- Perimylolysis is erosion over lingual surfaces of maxillary teeth due to reflux of gastric juices.
- Abfraction is the loss of tooth structure that results from repeated tooth flexure caused by occlusal stresses.

Internal Resorption

Appearance of pink-hued area on the crown of the tooth, which represents hyperplastic vascular pulp tissue filling the resorbed area and showing through remaining overlying tooth substance.

External Resorption

It arises as a result of a tissue reaction in the periodontal or pericoronal tissues. It may result due to periapical inflammation, reimplantation of teeth, tumors or cysts, excessive mechanical or occlusal forces, impacted teeth or due to idiopathic causes.

Discoloration of Teeth

- *Normal variation:* Primary teeth are comparatively whiter in color as compared to permanent teeth.
- *Physiological:* With advancing age color of the teeth becomes yellowish.
- Extrinsic discoloration can be seen due to:
  - *Bacterial stains:* Common cause, color can vary from green to brown-black to orange, common in children, involves labial surface of maxillary anterior teeth in gingival third.
  - *Excessive use of tobacco:* Brownish discoloration, involves lingual surface of maxillary incisors.
  - *Greenish discoloration:* Due to chromogenic bacteria, food containing chlorophyll, secondary to gingival hemorrhage.
  - *Large amalgam restorations:* Black discoloration of teeth.
  - *Medications:* Black pigmentation due to Fe and iodine, grayish-yellow to brown-black discoloration due to sulfides and silver nitrate, green

stain due to Cu/Ni, use of SnF produces black discoloration on labial aspect of anterior teeth and occlusal surface of posterior teeth and chlorhexidine mouth wash causes yellow-brown stains in interproximal areas.

- Intrinsic discoloration is seen in:
  - Erythroblastosis fetal is due to deposition of blood pigment in enamel and dentin of the developing teeth, which leads to green-brown or blue hue to teeth.
  - Erythropoietic porphyria which is a disorder of porphyrin metabolism, leads to reddish-brown discoloration that exhibits a red fluorescence when exposed to UV light.
  - Trauma produces yellow-dark gray discoloration of teeth due to deposition of degraded products of necrosed pulp.
  - Alkaptonuria leads to bluish-black discoloration termed as ochronosis.
  - Parkinson's disease causes bluish discoloration of dentition.
  - *Medications:* Tetracycline staining cause's bright yellow to dark brown discoloration of teeth. In UV light, teeth give bright yellow fluorescence. Minocycline HCl causes blue-gray discoloration of the incisal third.

Dental Caries

Dental caries is an irreversible microbial disease of the calcified tissues of the teeth, characterized by demineralization of the inorganic portion and destruction of the organic substance of the tooth, which often leads to cavitations. If there is a catch while exploration of the tooth, then it is considered as having decay. The role of the dentist is to not only find the known decay which can be seen easily but also to look for small pits which can lead to a future decay.

Clinical classification of caries is based on:

- According to morphology or site of lesion caries can be classified as pit or fissure caries, smooth surface caries and root caries.
- On the basis of dynamics in relation to the rate of caries progression they are classified as acute and chronic dental caries.
- Based on chronology, the caries can be either infant (rampant caries, nursing bottle caries) or adolescent caries.
- Based on the nature of attack caries can be primary or secondary (recurrent) caries or arrested caries.
- Based on the extent of caries they can be incipient (reversible) or cavitated (irreversible) lesions.
- According to the hard tissue involved caries may be affecting either enamel, dentin or cementum.

Initially, caries appears as opaque, chalky white areas over the teeth. Later brownish discoloration of teeth, followed by loss of tooth structure can be felt by the use of explorers. Caries diagnosis can be done by the following:

- Visual examination
- Tactile examination

- Conventional radiography
- Digital radiography
- Transillumination
- Digital Imaging Fibro Optic Transillumination
- UV illumination
- Near-IR light imaging
- Quantitative light fluorescence
- Diagnodent
- Endoscope/videoscope
- Ultrasound imaging
- Electronic caries meter
- Caries detecting dyes.

Occlusion

It refers to intercuspal relationship of teeth. In primary dentition there is generalized spacing in teeth which is normal, end-to-end relationship of distal surfaces of second molars, due to vertical inclination of lower anterior teeth anterior edge-to-edge relationship. In mixed dentition, primate spaces are present (mesial to maxillary canine and distal to mandibular canine); leeway space is present (M-D width of C+D+E > M-D width of 3+4+5) and freeway space is present.

In permanent teeth there are different types of occlusion seen in different individuals, which has been classified by Angle's as follows:

Angle's Class I malocclusion: Mesiobuccal cusp of maxillary first molar falls in mesiobuccal developmental groove of mandibular first molar. In case where first molar is missing then the mesial slope of maxillary first molar should coincide with the distal slope of mandibular first molar.

Angle's Class II malocclusion: Distobuccal cusp of maxillary first molar falls in mesiobuccal groove of mandibular first molar. In case where first molar is missing then the distal slope of maxillary canine should occlude with the mesial slope of mandibular canine. The maxillary central incisors are protruded while the maxillary lateral incisors may be retruded. It is further divided as division I and division II.

Angle's Class II subdivision where there is class I malocclusion on one side of molar relation and class II malocclusion on the other side of molar relation.

Angle's Class III malocclusion: Mesiobuccal cusp of maxillary first molar lies adjacent to distal aspect of mandibular first molar. The mandible is protruded anterior to the maxilla. There is spacing between the maxillary anteriors with protrusion.

Angle's Class III subdivision where, there is class III malocclusion on one side and class I malocclusion on the other side.

Canine guided occlusion is the one in which mesial incline of maxillary canine approximates distal incline of mandibular canine.

Examination of Swelling

Lumps and swellings in the mouth are common, but of diverse etiologies, and some represent malignant neoplasms. Important features to consider when making the provisional diagnosis of the cause of a lump or swelling include:

Position

The anatomical position should be defined and the proximity to other structures (e.g. teeth) noted. Midline lesions tend to be developmental in origin (e.g. torus palatinus). Bilateral lesions tend to be benign (e.g. sialosis: salivary swelling in alcoholism, diabetes or other conditions). Most neoplastic lumps are unilateral. Other similar or relevant changes elsewhere in the oral cavity should be noted.

Size

The size should always be measured and recorded. A diagram and photograph may be helpful.

Shape

Some swellings have a characteristic shape that may suggest the diagnosis: thus a parotid swelling often fills the space between the posterior border of the mandible and the mastoid process.

Color

Brown or black pigmentation may be due to a variety of causes such as a tattoo, naevus or melanoma. Purple or red may be due to a hemangioma, Kaposi's sarcoma or giant-cell lesion.

Temperature

The skin overlying acute inflammatory lesions, such as an abscess, or over a hemangioma, is frequently warm.

Tenderness

Inflammatory swellings such as an abscess are characteristically tender, although clearly palpation must be gentle to avoid excessive discomfort to the patient.

Discharge

Note any discharge from the lesion (e.g. clear fluid, pus, or blood), orifice, or sinus.

Movement

The swelling should be tested to determine if it is fixed to adjacent structures or the overlying skin/mucosa such as may be seen with a neoplasm.

Consistency

Palpation showing a hard (indurated) consistency may suggest a carcinoma. Palpation may cause the release of fluid (e.g. pus from an abscess) or cause the lesion to blanch (vascular) or occasionally cause a blister to appear (Nikolsky sign) or to expand. Sometimes palpation causes the patient pain (suggesting an inflammatory lesion). The swelling overlying a bony cyst may crackle (like an eggshell) when palpated or fluctuation may be elicited by detecting movement of fluid when the swelling is compressed. Palpation may disclose an underlying structure (e.g. the crown of a tooth under an eruption cyst) or show that the actual swelling is in deeper structures (e.g. submandibular calculus).

Surface Texture

The surface characteristics should be noted: papillomas have an obvious anemone-like appearance; carcinomas and other malignant lesions and deep fungal and other chromic infections tend to have a nodular surface and may ulcerate. Abnormal blood vessels suggest a neoplasm.

Ulceration

Some swellings may develop superficial ulceration such as squamous cell carcinoma. The character of the edge of the ulcer and the appearance of the ulcer base should also be recorded.

Margins

Ill-defined margins are frequently associated with malignancy, whereas clearly defined margins are suggestive of a benign lesion.

Number of Swellings

Multiple lesions suggest an infective or occasionally developmental, origin. Some conditions are associated with multiple swellings of a similar nature, e.g. neurofibromatosis.

The medical history should be fully reviewed, since some systemic disorders may be associated with intraoral or facial swellings. The nature of many lumps cannot be established without further investigation.

Examination of an Ulcer

Ulceration is a breach in the oral epithelium, which typically exposes nerve endings in the underlying lamina propria, resulting in pain or soreness, especially when eating spicy foods or citrus fruits. Patients vary enormously in the degree to which they suffer and complain of soreness in relation to oral ulceration. It is always important to exclude serious disorders such as oral cancer or other serious disease, but not all patients who complain of soreness have discernible organic disease. Conversely, some with serious disease have no pain. Even in those with detectable lesions, the level of complaint can vary enormously. Some patients with large ulcers complain little; others with minimal ulceration complain bitterly of discomfort. Sometimes there is a psychogenic influence.

Site

The anatomical position should be defined and the proximity to other structures (e.g. teeth) noted. Certain ulcers occur at specific site such as basal cell carcinoma is more common on the face; tuberculous/actinomycotic ulcers are common on the neck.

Size

The size should always be measured and recorded. A diagram and photograph may be helpful.

Shape

Some ulcers have a characteristic shape that may suggest the diagnosis.

Number

The number of ulcers should also be noted as they aid in diagnosis, such as recurrent aphthous major is characterized by 1–10 painful ulcers, while the number of ulcers in recurrent herpetiform ulcers may range up to 100.

Margin

It is the line of demarcation between normal and abnormal.

Edge

The edge is the portion in between the floor and margin of an ulcer. There are five main types of edges for ulcer:

1. *Sloping edge:* Usually, means the ulcer is superficial/shallow and has a good chance in healing. Healthy granulation tissue usually is pinkish, means it has a good vascularity. A healing epidermis is usually seen extending from the edge, over granulation tissue, either pale/pink in color (almost transparent). One example of such ulcer is venous ulcer.
2. *Punch-out edge:* It means there's rapid death over full thickness of tissue with minimal attempts of the body to repair it. A classical example is the ulcers seen in tertiary syphilis. Nowadays, ulcers with punch out edges are more commonly seen in neuropathic or peripheral arterial ischemic ulcers.
3. *Undermined edge:* It means the rate of destruction of the subcutaneous tissue is more rapid than the skin, causing the edge of ulcer to be undermined. Classical example, as it is rarely seen nowadays is tuberculous ulcers. Ulcers with undermined edge is more commonly seen in bedsores, pressure sores as the subcutaneous tissues are more susceptible towards pressure.

4. *Everted edge:* This means that over the edges of the ulcer, tissues are growing so rapid that it eventually overlaps the overlying skin. This is classically seen in squamous cell carcinoma.
5. *Rolled out edge:* The tissues over edges are growing slowly, which is usually pale/pink in color, with telengiectasis seen over the pearly edges. An ulcer with rolled edges is almost diagnostic of a rodent ulcer of basal cell carcinoma.

Discharge

Discharge from an ulcer can be serous, serosanguineous, sanguineous, or purulent. Sometimes, due to the formation of a coagulation discharge scab over an ulcer, it prevents you from examining the entire structure of ulcer. It is advised that the scab should be removed. The discharge may be serous, sanguineous or purulent.

Palpation may cause the release of fluid or cause the lesion to blanch. Sometimes palpation causes the patient pain or bleeding may be elicited by when the ulcer is examined. Palpation may disclose an underlying structure or show that the actual ulcer is involving the deeper structures. Measure the depth of an ulcer by millimeters and anatomically which structures are visible. Feel the base of the ulcer. Is it adherent to the underlying structure? (may be bone, periosteum, tendon in cases of osteomyelitis, malignancy). The floor of an ulcer usually is made up of granulation tissues or slough tissues. Sometimes, the underlying structures might be exposed, e.g. bones, tendons, etc. Some characteristic contents of the floor are able to provide you a hint to your diagnosis:

- Solid-brown, grayish tissue indicates full thickness death of tissue
- Slough tissue resembles a yellow-gray wash leather in syphilitic ulcers
- Unhealthy, bluish granulation tissue is observed in tuberculous ulcers
- Poor granulation tissue, with visible bones, tendons, periosteum is seen in ischemic ulcer.

Remember to palpate the regional lymph nodes. They may be enlarged and tender, if there are secondary metastatic deposits or any spreading infection. Assess local blood supply, local nerve supply and for evidence of previously healed ulcers. It is important to define the relation of the ulcer with surrounding structures, especially those deep to it. The examiner must try to ascertain whether the ulcer is adherent to deep structures.

The examination may confirm or refute a diagnosis suspected from the history and by adding this information a provisional diagnosis can be made. Summarize the history keeping in mind both the important positive and negative findings. Then provide a diagnosis, a differential diagnosis, a problem list, an investigation list, and a management plan.

Provisional Diagnosis

At the onset of diagnostic investigations, provisional diagnosis is made. This implies that available information favors a certain diagnosis but additional diagnostic studies will be conducted to substantiate this impression.

Differential Diagnosis

When different diseases are held responsible for the patient's signs/symptoms, differential diagnosis is made, one by one disease are ruled out according to the signs/symptoms produced.

Final Diagnosis

This indicates that a definitive diagnosis has been made on the basis of all necessary observations and laboratory investigations.

Ask the patient what they want out of their visit and which problems are most important. Tell the patient what will happen next. Check that the patient understands and agrees the management plan before seeking senior help.

6

Investigations

Introduction

Laboratory examinations are an important and at times deemed necessary for the diagnostic process. Ordering and interpreting diagnostic tests are fundamental skills. However, evidence indicates that many of us are poorly trained in this vital area. Studies have shown that physicians commonly order more laboratory tests than required, use them for the wrong purposes, and ignore or misinterpret their results. While these errors have obvious implications for the quality of patient care, there are large socioeconomic implications as well. These investigations when implied for the right purpose provide information that helps to make early and a more definitive diagnosis which may lead to better therapeutic outcomes. The routine examinations include radiographs, biopsies or cultures and it is rarely necessary for the dental practitioners to obtain special examinations. Laboratory investigations are not routinely used by the dentist; and this should not imply that the dentist that they lack knowledge of various basic laboratory examinations or are not familiar with these procedures.

Investigations are the extension of physical examination where tissue; blood and other specimens obtained from patients are subjected to microscopic, biochemical and microbiological examination. These are necessary in diagnosing and managing a few complicated conditions. A laboratory test alone may not establish the nature of the oral lesion, but when combined with the information obtained from the patients' history and physical examination; it will frequently establish or confirm the diagnostic impression. These are useful in determining the systemic manifestations of oral infections and vice-versa. Patients may be unaware of some underlying systemic diseases like diabetes mellitus, tuberculosis, syphilis, anemia and cancers; which may be present for many years without the patient knowing them. These routine laboratory investigations may provide useful information to make the patient aware of the underlying disease and/or condition. Dental practitioners must therefore, be aware of the investigations, required to establish diagnosis of general medical and surgical problems; and of the principles of treatment, including drug prescriptions. They should also obtain verbal and written informed consent wherever required, for invasive or risky procedures.

The rationale behind this chapter is to improve the quality of care you offer to your patients while decreasing its cost. Both aims can be achieved by a rational approach to diagnostic test ordering and interpretation. After reading this chapter, you should have an understanding of the probabilistic nature of diagnosis and its implications for ordering and interpreting laboratory tests, the basic operating characteristics that define a laboratory test: reliability (precision), accuracy, sensitivity, specificity, and predictive value, various purposes for which laboratory tests are ordered (diagnosis, monitoring therapy, and screening) and the operating characteristics for each purpose.

Several characteristics of tests are crucial to their interpretation. Two of these operating characteristics enable you to judge the test *per se:* reliability and accuracy. The other characteristics enable you to judge a test with respect to how its results affect your diagnostic probabilities: sensitivity, specificity, and predictive value (positive and negative).The reliability (or precision) of a test is a measure of reproducibility obtained by running the test many times on the same specimen. An unreliable test is one that yields results that vary widely due to chance or technical error. Such tests are therefore very difficult to interpret because day-to-day variation in a given test may be due to something other than a true change in the patient's condition. Such changes in a reliable test, in contrast, are more likely to reflect true patient change. Test accuracy reflects the degree to which the test result reflects the 'true' value. It is important to realize that test reliability and accuracy may vary independently of one another. A test may be inaccurate but totally reliable.

Since the advent of multichannel chemistry laboratory equipment, it has become fashionable 'routinely' to order laboratory tests on every patient admitted to the hospital. The tests usually include a complete blood count, coagulation profile, urine analysis, serum electrolytes, some combination of serum chemistries, an electrocardiogram and a chest X-ray. These tests are ordered routinely, that is without regard to the actual admitting diagnosis or underlying probabilities. The two reasons usually cited to justify this process are that these tests are helpful in screening for asymptomatic disease and that they are useful in defining a 'database,' a baseline set of data in the light of which future changes can be evaluated. Admission or database testing should never be routine; instead, it should be tailored to the differing needs of individual or selected groups of patients over time.

The diagnostic tests can be divided as:

- *Chair-side investigations:* They are the simple and rapid procedures that require inexpensive equipment and no specialized training. These investigations include: Pulp vitality tests, plaque disclosing agents, caries detecting dyes, Toluidine blue and Lugol's iodine staining, salivary flow test, diagnostic nerve blocking techniques, culture and sensitivity test and diascopic examination.
- *Laboratory procedures:* They include simple tests that can be carried out easily in an office or a clinic, but require trained medical technician and a especially equipped laboratory. They comprise hematological, histopathological, biochemical, microbiological, immunological and serological tests.

Laboratory procedures can be further divided as:

- Screening Tests
- Diagnostic Tests

The object of the use of diagnostic tests for screening is to detect disease in its earliest, presymptomatic state when, presumably, it is less widespread and more easily treated or cured. These simple and inexpensive tests should be sensitive. The sensitivity of a test refers to the proportion of patients with a given disease who have a positive test. On the other hand, diagnostic tests are supporting tests to confirm the diagnosis, as they are more elaborate and specific tests. These tests are specific. The specificity of a test refers to the proportion of patients without the disease who have a negative test.

The various investigations useful in dentistry are discussed in the following section.

Plaque Disclosing Agents

A disclosing agent is a liquid, tablet or lozenge preparation containing a dye or other similar coloring agent used for the identification of bacterial plaque. This is a valuable aid for detecting the site of plaque, demonstrating the presence of plaque to patient, as a personalized educating aid for the patients to determine the efficacy of home care procedures and self-monitoring them, detecting irregular and rough surfaces that are susceptible to take up stains and in research studies.

These agents can be applied using a cotton pellet and applying on all the tooth surfaces or rinsing and swishing the solution over all the teeth or by chewing the tablet or wafer and swishing it for 30–60 seconds, followed by rinsing.

Few of the commonly used agents are as follows:

- *Iodine preparations:* Skinner's iodine solution and diluted tincture of iodine
- *Mercurochrome preparations:* 5% mercurochrome solution and flavored mercurochrome disclosing solution
- Bismark brown
- Merbromin
- *Erythrosine:* FD and C (Federal Food Drug and Cosmetic Act) Red no. 3/ no. 28
- *Fast green:* FD and C green no. 3
- *Fluorescein:* FD and C yellow no. 8 (used with special UV source to make it visible)
- *Two-tone solution:* FD and C blue no. 1 and FD and C red no. 3. It mainly stains older, subgingival plaque blue and newer, supragingival plaque red.
- Basic fuchsin.

Caries Detecting Dyes

Dyes uptake by enamel lesions would be very advantageous since it would allow lesions to be visualized at an early stage. Dyes used for caries detection are:

- 0.5% basic fuchsin
- 1% acid red

0.5% basic fuchsin has carcinogenic potential and stains the unaffected coronal dentin, so it is replaced by 1% acid red.

Pulp Vitality Tests

Pulp vitality tests are widely used as diagnostic aids in assessing the degree of pulpal disease. These tests do not quantify the disease, nor do they measure the health of the pulp, but the pathological status of the pulp. A delta fibers are involved in cold test, dentin sensitivity and electric pulp vitality tests and C fibers are involved in heat test.

Uses of Pulp Vitality Testing

- Prior to restorative or orthodontic procedures, to know the status of the teeth, even if teeth are asymptomatic
- Diagnosis of oral pain
- Investigation of radiolucent areas present at the apical part
- Assessment of traumatized teeth
- Assessment of teeth, which have been pulp capped or which have required deep restorations.
- Assessment of anesthesia.

Various types of pulp vitality tests are:

- Thermal tests
- Electrical pulp testing
- Test cavity
- Anesthesia test
- Bite test
- Pulp oximetry
- Transillumination
- Laser Doppler Flowmetry
- Staining
- Others.

Thermal Pulp Tests

These tests are based on one of the most common symptoms associated with symptomatic inflamed pulp, i.e. pain elicited by thermal stimulation. When pulp responds abnormally to thermal stimulation, it indicates that the pulp is not in a state of good health. They are of further two types: heat test and cold test.

- *Cold test:* It is the most commonly used test and can be done in a number of ways as follows:
  - The most commonly used method is to **spray with cold air**.
  - *Ice-sticks:* These can be prepared by freezing water in plastic covers from hypodermic needles. Ice-stick is applied immediately to middle third of facial surface of crown of tooth or on any exposed metal surface of

the crown and kept in contact for 5 seconds or until patient starts to feel the pain. Rubber dam isolation is must when using ice-sticks as the melting ice may run over the gingival or adjacent teeth, thus reporting a false positive test.

- *Cold water bath:* The tooth is isolated with rubber dam and bathed with ice water from a syringe for 5 seconds. This elicits a most accurate response as, simultaneously all surfaces of the tooth are cooled. Similarly, an ice piece can be wrapped in a wet guage and applied to the tooth to assess the vitality.
- *Ethyl chloride:* It is available as compressed spray. However, it is no longer recommended as it has been found to be less effective than carbon dioxide snow or dichlorodifluromethane (Freon). The recently available material is 1,1,1,2 tetra fluromethane, which is the non-chloroflurocarbon refrigerant R-134 a. It is sprayed onto a cotton pallet or swab, and kept in contact for 5 seconds or until the patient reports any pain, on the middle 1/3rd of facial surface of crown of tooth.
- *Carbon dioxide snow:* It is formed into sticks, is extremely cold and is the most effective method of eliciting a response in vital teeth. The carbon dioxide is released into a special syringe where it forms the snow. It is applied immediately to the middle third of facial surface of crown of tooth or on any exposed metal surface of the crown and kept in contact for a few seconds or until patient begins to feel pain. It can penetrate full coverage restoration and can elicit a pulpal reaction to the cold due to its very low temperature.

- *Heat test:* It is most advantageous when the patient complains of intense pain during intake of hot solid or liquid food. It can be done using various methods such as:
  - *Warm sticks of temporary stopping:* In this gutta-percha stick is used. The teeth to be tested are coated with a lubricant such as a light coating of petroleum jelly to prevent the gutta-percha from adhering to the tooth. Gutta-percha is warmed over the flame until it becomes soft and applied to middle third of facial surface of crown. Prolonged duration of application has been found to increase the temperature at the pulpo-dentinal junction, and is therefore likely to damage the pulp.
  - **Hot burnisher, hot compound** or any other heated instrument may also be used.
  - *Hot water bath:* The isolated tooth is bathed with warm water from a syringe to determine the pulpal response. Temperature is gradually increased if no response is obtained rather than producing unnecessary pain by beginning with excessively hot water bath. This gives most accurate response but it is time consuming. It is useful for teeth with porcelain or full-coverage restorations.
  - **Frictional heat by rotating polishing rubber disc** against the tooth surface may also be used.
  - **Nd:YAG laser** has also been employed for thermal pulp testing.

Mild, transitory response to stimulation shows a normal pulp, while an absence of response indicated necrosis of pulp. An exaggerated or delayed response indicates irreversible pulpitis. However, sometimes a false positive response may be elicited owing to the following reasons:

- Excessive calcification may interfere with nerve conduction.
- Recently erupted teeth with immature apex are not capable of transmitting the pain due to incompletely developed plexus of Rashkow.
- Recent trauma to the nerve supply or presence of inflammatory exudates around the apex also interferes with nerve conduction.
- Patients taking premedication such as analgesics or tranquilizers.

In the young permanent tooth, heat test is more reliable than cold test as C fibers are more and very little A delta fibers are present in young permanent tooth. Heat tests incite the C fibers. During the heat test, the heat is transmitted to the body of the pulp, resulting in expansion of blood vessels and an increase in pulpal pressure, which in turn incites the C fibers.

Electric Pulp Tests

These tests use electric excitation to stimulate A delta sensory fibers within the pulp. A positive response indicates that there are vital sensory fibers within the pulp, but does not provide any information about health or integrity of pulp. No response indicates nonvital pulp or pulpal necrosis.

Procedure: The patient should be informed of the nature of the test. Teeth to be tested should be dried and adequate electric current contact should be made between the tooth and electrode. The electrode should be placed on sound tooth structure. The electrode should not touch or be in proximity to the gingiva, as contact with gingival tissue may result in a false positive response. An excessively applied stimulus is likely to result in a false positive test due to leakage. Electrical conduction through proximal inlays and continuous bridgework should also be avoided. Teeth with full gold, porcelain or acrylic coverage cannot be tested with an electrical stimulus. Each tooth should be tested 2–3 times and average reading should be recorded. Pulp tests should be supported with the findings from history and clinical examination.

Various types of electric pulp testers that are in use are as follows:

- Analytic technology pulp tester
- Vitapulp pulp tester
- Ritter pulp tester
- Parkell dentotest vitalometer
- Digilog pulp tester
- Neotest automatic digital pulp tester.

In certain cases a false positive response may be observed due to:

- Patient's anxiety
- Saliva conducting stimulus to gingival
- Metallic restorations conducting stimulus to adjacent teeth
- Liquefactive necrosis conducting the stimulus to attachment apparatus.

Whereas, in certain cases a false negative response may be seen due to:

- Patients taking premedication such as analgesics or tranquilizers
- Recently erupted teeth with immature apex
- Recently traumatized teeth
- Poor contact with teeth
- Inadequate contact media
- Partial necrosis of vital pulp, which is sometimes indicated as total necrosis
- Calcified canals
- Patients with high pain threshold
- Poor battery or electrical deficiency of pulp testers
- Teeth with extensive restorations or pulp protecting bases under the restorations.

Fuss and associates in an *in vivo* study comparing tooth vitality, produced a positive vitality response of 98.7% with dichlorodifluoromethane, 97.4% with carbon dioxide snow, 94.8% with electric pulp tests, 53.2% with ethyl chloride and 32.5% with ice.

Test Cavity

This test is performed when other methods of diagnosis have been inconclusive. The test cavity is made by drilling through the enamel-dentin junction of an unanesthetized tooth. The drilling is done with high speed number 1 or 2 round burs, with adequate air and water coolant. Sensitivity or pain felt by the patient is an indication of pulp vitality, no endodontic treatment is indicated. Sedative cement is then placed in cavity and search for source of pain continues. If no pain is felt, the cavity preparation is continued until the pulp chamber is reached. If pulp is completely necrotic endodontic treatment can be continued painlessly in many cases without anesthesia.

Anesthetic Testing

When the patient is unable to specify the site of pain and other tests have been inconclusive, this test is obviously a last resort. A single tooth is anesthetized at a time until pain disappears and is localized to a specific tooth. Using either infiltration or intra ligament injection, inject the most posterior tooth in area suspected of being the cause of pain. If pain persists when tooth has been fully anesthetized, anesthetize the next tooth mesial to it and continue to do so until pain disappears. If the source of pain cannot be determined, whether maxillary or mandibular teeth, an inferior alveolar nerve block is should be given. Cessation of pain naturally indicates involvement of mandibular tooth and localization of specific tooth is done by intraligament injection. This test has advantage over 'Test cavity' during which iatrogenic damage is possible.

Bite Test or Wedging

This test is helpful when the patient complains of pain on mastication. Tooth is sensitive to biting if pulpal necrosis has reached the periodontal ligament space or a crack is present in the tooth. The patient is asked to bite on a hard object such as cotton swab, tooth pick or orange wood stick with suspected and contralateral tooth. Tooth sloth is a commercially available device for bite test with a small concave surface on its top. This is placed in contact with the cusp to be tested and patient is asked to bite. Pain on biting may indicate a fractured tooth. This technique helps the clinician identify both vertical crown fracture and cuspal shear fracture that may not involve the pulp.

Pulp Oximetry

This is a noninvasive device which is widely used for recording blood oxygen saturation levels during administration of intravenous anesthesia. Increased acidity and metabolic rate produced by inflammation cause deoxygenating of Hb and change the oxygen saturation of blood. A pulse oximeter uses a probe containing a diode that emits light in two wavelengths: red light-approximately 660 nm and infrared light-approximately 850 nm, which is received by photo detector diode, connected to a microprocessor. It compares the ratio of amplitudes of the transmitted infrared with red light and uses this information, together with known absorption curves for oxygenated and deoxygenated Hb to determine the oxygen saturation levels.

By monitoring changes in oxygen saturation pulp oximetry may be able to detect pulpal inflammation or partial necrosis in teeth that are still. It is especially useful in cases of traumatic injury to the tooth, where blood supply remains intact but nerve supply is damaged. A distinctive advantage of this technique is its objectivity and lack of dependence on sensory response which eliminates the need for application of an unpleasant stimulus to the patient.

Laser Doppler Flowmetry

Vitality of pulp depends on blood supply to the pulp. This is shown by laser Doppler flowmetry test. The technique depends on the Doppler principle where a low power light from a monochromatic laser beam of known wavelength along a fiberoptic cable is directed to the tooth surface, where the light passes along the direction of enamel prisms and dentinal tubules to the pulp. Moving red blood cells cause frequency of laser beam to be Doppler shifted and some of the light to be back scattered out of tooth in a photo detector. Some light is reflected back to the flowmeter where the frequency broadened light, together with laser light from static tissue, is photo detected for strength of signal and pulsatility. Laser Doppler flowmetry is complicated by the fact the laser beam must interact with moving cells within the pulpal vasculature. The position on crown of tooth and location of pulp with in tooth causes variations in pulpal blood flow measurements.

The blood flow measured by this technique is termed as 'flux', which is proportional to the product of average speed of blood cells and their concentration. The blood flux level in vital teeth is much higher than non-vital teeth.

This test can be used in young children since it produces no noxious stimuli. It is an objective and accurate test for checking pulp vitality. However, it cannot be used in patients who refrain from moving or if tooth to be tested cannot be stabilized. It is an expensive test which requires higher technical skills. Medications used by cardiovascular patients may affect the blood flow to the pulp.

Transillumination

In this method fibroptic illuminating device is used whereby light is passed through a finely drawn glass or plastic fibers by a process known as total internal reflection. A bore light or fibro-optic hand piece may be used for this purpose. Normally, the fibroptic light will illuminate the crown of intact tooth uniformly, but if a fracture exists, the light will illuminate the side of the crown that contacts. However, portion of the crown on opposite side of fracture will remain dark. Composite curing lights are not recommended, because they are excessively bright and despite the fracture may illuminate the entire crown. If tooth contains restoration it may necessary to remove it to expose the fracture line.

Staining

In staining method methylene blue or erythrosine dye is used. This is indicated in subtle coronal fracture that might otherwise escape detection.

Other available tests are:
- Dual wavelength spectrophotometry
- Measurement of temperature of tooth surface
- Plethysmography
- Detection of interleukin-1β
- Xenon-133
- Hughes probeye camera
- Gas desaturation
- Radiolabeled microspheres
- Electromagnetic flowmetry.

Toludine Blue and Lugol's Iodine Staining

Both the stains are used as additional aids in assessing high-risk patients and suspicious oral lesions. Toludine blue which has been used effectively as the nuclear stain because of its binding with DNA is a metachromatic dye of the Thiazine group. It is used for detection of oral precancerous and malignant lesions such as: hyperplasia, keratosis, inflammation and lichen planus. Toludine blue rinses are used for screening high-risk patients who may have asymptomatic malignant lesions of oral cavity. Toludine blue does not show tumor present beneath the normal epithelium. The dye uptake also assists the clinician in the evaluation by marking lesion margins; however with benign lesions the dye uptake at the margins is in contrast to the diffuse marginal patterns associated with dysplastic or malignant lesions. This false positive dye uptake by benign oral ulcerative lesions confuses rather than aid the dental practitioners in the judgments. Filiform papillae retain the dye; due to high protein synthesis rate.

Lugol's iodine solution produces a brown black stain by reaction of iodine with glycogen. Iodine does not interfere with the histological evaluation as it is removed by fixation in alcohol and formaldehyde in the preparation of biopsy specimen. Normal tissue stain brown, but proliferating epithelium would be unstained or poorly stained. When both stains are used they show better specificity (73.3–92.9%) and sensitivity (93.5–97.8%) than toludine blue used alone. Lesions which are studied using both the stains are: granulation tissue, benign keratosis, dysplasia, carcinoma *in situ*, squamous cell carcinoma, lichen planus and mucoepidermoid carcinoma.

Salivary Flow Test

- Normal salivary flow rate is 1.0–1.5 L/day
- *Flow rate of unstimulated saliva:* 0.3 mL/min
- *Flow rate of stimulated saliva:* 1.5–2.0 mL/min

The orifices of parotid duct are inspected and palpated. Parotid papilla and Stenson's duct should be palpated with index finger of one hand placed inside the mouth and of other hand placed outside the cheek. Inflammation of parotid papilla, together with expression of turbid saliva from a duct and signs and symptoms of swelling and pain in parotid region suggests inflammation of parotid gland. Inflammation of incisive papilla, expression of purulent saliva and the presence of a hard mass in the Stenson's duct suggest a sialolith in the duct. A tumor or neoplasm may be suspected when there is enlargement of the gland with or without visible signs or symptoms of changes in saliva especially in the absence of systemic symptoms.

The factors such as degree of hydration, position of the body, exposure to light, previous stimulation, circadian rhythm and certain drugs such as antipsychotics, antidepressants and anticonvulsants directly affect the unstimulated salivary flow rate in healthy subjects. When body water is reduced by 8%, the salivary flow rate decreases, whereas hyperhydration increases the flow rate. On standing flow increases and on lying down it tends to decrease. Flow increases during late afternoon and drops to almost zero during sleep.

The gender, age and weight of the patient, size of the gland, mental stress, thought and sight of food and functional stimulation also affect the unstimulated salivary flow rate but not to a great extent.

However, age and gland size directly affect the stimulated salivary flow. As the gland size increases, the flow also increases and vice-versa. There is a reduction in the proportion of secretory cells with age and elderly people receive more medication. This leads to a greater tendency for reduction in salivary flow. Flow increases just prior to and during vomiting. Also the nature of the stimuli affects the flow rate, such as acidic stimuli and unilateral chewing increase the flow on the side of chewing.

Xerostomia

Decrease in secretion of salivary flow is xerostomia. When unstimulated flow rate is less than 0.1 mL/min and stimulated flow is less than 0.5 mL/min the condition is referred to as xerostomia. It is not a disease but can be symptom of certain other diseases. It may be caused by the following factors:

1. *Water/metabolite loss:* Impaired water intake, loss of water through skin, blood loss, emesis, diarrhea, polyurea and protein malnutrition lead to decreased salivary flow rate.
2. **Damage to salivary glands** due to therapeutic irradiation to head and neck and autoimmune conditions such as: Sjögren's syndrome, graft versus host disease, systemic lupus erythomatosis and rheumatoid arthritis also decrease the flow.
3. **Interference with the neural transmission** due to certain drugs, autonomic dysfunction, conditions affecting the central nervous system (CNS), psychogenic disorders, trauma and decrease in mastication also decrease the salivary flow rate.

Ptyalism is defined as increase in salivary flow. It is more commonly observed in patients wearing new prosthodontic appliances and orthodontic appliances, during first trimester of pregnancy, patients with psychological disorders and primary herpetic and other infections. However, with the resolution of the underlying problem it usually disappears.

Diagnostic Nerve Blocking

For the diagnosis of masticatory pain and nonmasticatory myofacial pain disorders skillful analgesic blocking of masticatory muscles, i.e. temporalis, masseter, lateral pterygoid and medial pterygoid and muscles of maxillofacial region such as, trapezius, sternocleidomastoid, diagastric and splenius capitis as well as anesthetizing the temporomandibular joint (TMJ) are especially useful. The clinician should have sufficient knowledge of the anatomical landmarks, technique and other related information. However, these blocks should not be used in severe acute cases of muscle injury, trauma, or pain, patients who are allergies to the anesthetics used for the procedure, patients with cellulitis, active bleeding difficulties, diathesis, or on anticoagulant therapy.

Antibiotic Sensitivity Test

It is necessary to identify the most effective antibiotic against a particular strain of bacteria. Very few dental clinics have the necessary equipment for collecting a specimen for culture media. Hence, the specimen obtained at the dental clinic is sent immediately to the laboratory or the patient is referred to the concerned laboratory or physician. These tests are of the following two types:

1. *Diffusion test:* Filter paper discs of 6 mm in diameter are used. After overnight incubation, the degree of sensitivity is determined by measuring zones of inhibition of growth around the discs. Growth will be inhibited around the discs containing antibiotics to which bacteria are susceptible

but not around those to which it is resistant. The results are reported as sensitive, moderately sensitive or resistant to different drugs.

2. *Dilution test:* It is of 2 types- tube dilution method and agar dilution method. Tube dilution method uses serial dilutions of drug in broth that are taken in tubes and a standardized suspension of test *Bacterium* is inoculated. After overnight incubation, the 'minimum inhibitory concentration' is read by noting the lowest concentration of drug that inhibits growth. The 'minimum bactericidal concentration' can be estimated by sub-culturing from lowest concentration of drug that kills the *Bacterium.*

   In the agar dilution method several strains are tested at the same time. The serial dilutions of drug are prepared in agar and poured into plates. The advantage is that many strains can be inoculated on each plate containing an antibiotic dilution.

Diascopic Examination

In this technique the pressure is applied to the suspected vascular lesions to visualize the evacuation of coloration, a finding that supports the fact that patent blood filled spaces constitutes the lesion. If compression fails to evacuate the pigmentation, the lesion is extravasated blood or some other type of intrinsic or extrinsic pigment that has been deposited in the tissues, such as hemangiomas.

Hematological Investigations

When a patient reports with the complain of bleeding from the gums, weakness, inability to do work, pallor of oral mucous membrane and tongue and excessive bleeding from the extraction site, blood investigations are advised. Hematological investigations play a very significant role in the diagnosis of various diseases. Blood investigations comprise the following:

1. Determination of hemoglobin
2. Packed cell volume
3. Erythrocyte sedimentation rate
4. Erythrocyte constants
5. Examination of blood smear
6. Red blood cell count
7. White blood cell count
8. Differential leukocyte count
9. Absolute eosinophil count
10. Reticulocyte count
11. Platelet count
12. Bleeding and clotting time
13. Clot retraction time
14. Prothrombin time
15. Partial thromboplastin time and activated partial thromboplastin time
16. Capillary fragility test
17. Bone marrow aspiration

18. Sickle cell preparation
19. Hemoglobin electrophoresis
20. Serum iron and total iron binding capacity
21. Serum fibrinogen.

Determination of Hemoglobin

Hemoglobin (Hb) is the protein contained in RBC's that is responsible for delivery of oxygen to the tissues. To ensure adequate tissue oxygenation, a sufficient hemoglobin level must be maintained. Hemoglobin concentration is expressed as grams of Hb per deciliter of blood. It is measured commonly to obtain information about circulating RBS's and the amount of oxygen carrying substance they contain, thereby providing information similar to that given by the total red blood cell count and hematocrit. The normal values of Hb are as under:

Infants	15–25 g/dL
Children (up to 1 year)	11–14 g/dL
Children (10–12 years)	11.5–14.5 g/dL
Men	14–18 g/dL
Women	12–16 g/dL
Pregnant women	11–14 g/dL

Decreased hemoglobin is observed in pregnancy, anemia (various types), excessive bleeding, erythropoietin deficiency (from kidney disease), lead poisoning, malnutrition, nutritional deficiencies of iron, folate, vitamin B_{12}, vitamin B_6, over hydration, red blood cell destruction associated with transfusion reaction.

Increased hemoglobin is observed when there is loss of body fluid in severe diarrhea and vomiting, hypoxia, congenital heart disease, emphysema, polycythemia vera, chronic obstructive pulmonary disease (COPD), high altitude, smoking and thalassemia minor.

Various methods of hemoglobin estimation are as under:

- Sahli's method
- Cyanmethemoglobin method
- Oxyhemoglobin method
- Alkaline hematin method
- Halden's carboxyhemoglobin method
- Gasometric determination method
- Specific gravity method
- Photometric method.

Determination of Packed Cell Volume or Hematocrit

The hematocrit measures the volume of red blood cells compared to the total blood volume (red blood cells and plasma). Packed cell volume is the amount of packed RBC's, following centrifugation, expressed as percentage of the total blood volume. The premature ventricular contractions (PCV) increases in anemias and hydremia. Decreased PVC is observed in polycythemia, dehydration, emphysema and congenital heart disease. It can be determined by:

- Macrohematocrit method/Wintrobe's method
- Microhematocrit method
- Electronic counters.

At birth	54%
2 months	42%
1–2 years	36%
4 years	37%
8 years	39%
12 years	40%
Male	40–54%
Female	36–48%

Erythrocyte Sedimentation Rate

It is the rate at which the red cell fall. Erythrocyte sedimentation rate (ESR) determination is useful to check the progress of the disease and not the diagnosis of any specific diseases. It increased in cases of tuberculosis, chronic infections, rheumatic fever, multiple myeloma, Kala-azar, oral submucous fibrosis, anemia, increased temperature, malignancies and rheumatoid arthritis. During pregnancy ESR increases after 3 months and returns to normal in about 3–4 weeks after delivery.

Erythrocyte sedimentation rate (ESR) decreases in polycythemia, sickle cell anemia, hypochromic anemia, congestive cardiac failure, severe dehydration, whooping cough, cholera and acute gastritis.

It can be measured using:

- Westergren's method, where the normal values recorded after 1 hour are:
  - *In newborn:* 0–5 mm
  - *Children:* 3–10 mm
  - *Male:* 0–15 mm
  - *Female:* 0–20 mm
- Wintrobe's method, where the normal values in males range from 0–9 mm after 1 hour and 0–20 mm after 1 hour in females.

Determination of Erythrocyte Indices (Wintrobe's Constants)

Mean corpuscular volume (MCV), mean corpuscular hemoglobin (MCH), and mean corpuscular hemoglobin concentration (MCHC) were first introduced by Wintrobe in 1929 to define the size (MCV) and hemoglobin content (MCH, MCHC) of red blood cells. These values are useful in elucidating the etiology of anemias. These indices can be calculated if the values of hemoglobin, hematocrit (packed cell volume), and red blood cell count are known. With the general availability of electronic cell counters, red cell indices are now automatically measured in all blood count determinations. Anemias may be classified based on their etiology (e.g. hemolytic, hemorrhagic, etc.), erythropoietic response (e.g. hypoproliferative, ineffective), or cell morphology (e.g. macrocytic, microcytic-hypochromic). Red cell indices are valuable in the morphologic classification of anemias. The most commonly calculated indices are:

- *Mean cell volume (MCV):* The normal range varies from 77 to 93 fl. It increases in macrocytic anemia and a decrease is observed during microcytic anemia.
- *Mean corpuscular hemoglobin (MCH):* The normal value ranges from 27 to 32 pg. A increased value is observed in macrocytic anemia, while in hypochromia the value of MCH decreases.
- *Mean corpuscular hemoglobin concentration (MCHC):* The normal value ranges from 30 to 35 g/dL. It is the portion of average red blood cells containing hemoglobin. An increased value is observed in hypochromic anemia, while the value decreases in spherocytosis.
- *Color index (CI):* It denotes the ratio of hemoglobin to RBC. It is an insignificant index, because normal range of RBC is very wide.

Examination of the Peripheral Blood Smear

Examination of the peripheral blood smear should be considered, along with review of the results of peripheral blood counts and red blood cell indices, an essential component of the initial evaluation of all patients with hematologic disorders. The examination of blood films stained with Wright's stain frequently provides important clues in the diagnosis of anemias and various disorders of leukocytes and platelets that show certain significant changes in the peripheral blood smear.

Example of various types of erythrocytes and the conditions where they are present	
Microcytes	Chlorosis, Iron deficiency anemia, after chronic hemorrhage, most cases of secondary anemia
Macrocytes	Pernicious anemia, sprue, pregnancy, tropical malnutrition, megaloblastic anemia
Anisocytes	Severe anemia
Acanthocytes	A beta lipoproteinemia and in the 'spur cell anemia' associated with severe alcoholic liver disease
Poikilocytes	Severe anemia, iron deficiency anemia, after hemorrhage
Elliptocytes	Hereditary elliptocytosis, thalassemia and myelofibrosis, iron deficiency and hyperspleníc states
Echinocytes	Pyruvate kinase deficiency of erythrocytes, uremia, carcinomas, immediately after the transfusion of aged or metabolically depleted blood

Hypochromic cells	Hypochromic anemia
Leptocytes	Thalassemic disorders and with obstructive liver disease
Spherocytes	Hereditary spherocytosis, burns, ABO incompatibility
Stomatocytes	Alcoholics and in the rare disorder of hereditary stomatocytosis
Target cells	Liver disease with jaundice, thalassemia, sickle cell anemia, post splenectomy state, hereditary spherocytosis, Hb-c disease
Sickle cells and dense, deformed poikilocytes ('irreversibly sickled cells')	Sickle cell anemia, hemoglobin SC disease, hemoglobin S-thalassemia, hemoglobin C-Harlem
Burr cells	Artifact, uremia, splenectomy
Spur cells	Spur cell anemia, anorexia nervosa, Abetalipoproteinemia
Schizocytes	Microangiopathic hemolytic anemias, disseminated intravascular coagulation
Howell jolly bodies	Megaloblastic anemia, after splenectomy, Acholuric jaundice
Cabot ring	Pernicious anemia, Leukemia, lead poisoning
Basophilic stippling	Anemia due to chronic lead poisoning, Aplastic anemia, thalassemia
Boat shaped cells	Hbsc disease
Heinz bodies	G6PD deficiency

Examples of various types of leukocytes and conditions where they are present	
Auer bodies	Acute myleoid leukemia
Dohle bodies	Severe infections, burns, during pregnancy, after cytotoxic chemotherapy (particularly with cyclophosphamide), with the May–Heggelin anomaly
Hypersegmentation	Macrocytic anemia, myelodysplasia or myeloproliferative disorders
Hyposegmentation	AML, severe infections, toxic states, hereditary disorders
Pelger–Hüet cells	Neutrophilic granulocytic dysplasia
Smudge cells	Chronic lymhocytic leukemia
Toxic granulation	Severe bacterial infections, in some hereditary disorders
Vacuoles	Severe infections, burns, chemical poisoning, in malignancy

Red Blood Cell Count

The red blood cell (RBC) count increases due to hemoconcentration because burns, cholera, in central cyanotic states as seen in chronic heart disease, polycythemia and emphysema. It decreases in old age, pregnancy and anemia.

RBC can be measured by using electronic counters or visual counting using the Neubauer's chamber.

- Normal range:
  - *At birth:* 6.5–7.5 millions/mm^3
  - *Males:* 4.5–6.5 millions/mm^3
  - *Females:* 3.8–5.8 millions/mm^3

Total Leukocyte Count

It increases in the following cases:

- Physiological leucocytosis: exercise, digestion, fear and pain
- Acute and chronic infections
- Polycythemia
- Leukemia

Decreased total leukocyte count (TLC) is noticed in influenza, measles, malignant neutropenia, respiratory tract infections, catarrhal jaundice, typhoid and paratyphoid fevers and reaction to certain drugs, such as amidopyrine, barbiturates and sulfonamides.

At birth	10,000–25,000/cumm
1-3 years	6,000–18,000/cumm
4-7 years	6,000–15,000/cumm
8-12 years	4,500–13,500/cumm
Adults	4,000–11,000/cumm

Differential Leukocyte Count

Differential leukocyte count is the percent distribution of various white cells in the peripheral blood. The various leukocytes, their normal range and clinical significance is as under:

Leukocyte (Normal range)	*Increases*	*Decreases*
Neutrophils (40–75% 3000–7000/cumm)	*Physiological:* Exercise, pregnancy, neonatal period *Pharmacological:* Epinephrine, and steroid therapy *Pathological:* Infection with pyogenic organisms, non-infective inflammation, neoplasm, leukemia, myocardial infarction, pulmonary embolism, hemorrhages, trauma and following surgery	Starvation and debility Infections and toxemia in old people Infections like typhoid, measles, malaria, kala-azar, hepatitis, influenza, etc., Hypersplenism, bone marrow failure *Pharmacological:* Due to certain drugs such as phenothiazines, phenylbutazone, and allopurinol

Contd...

Contd...

Eosinophils (1–6% 40–400/cumm)	*Allergic:* Hay fever, urticaria, asthma, food sensitivity. *Parasitic infections:* Hookworm, ameobiasis, filariasis, etc. *Collagen diseases:* Rheumatoid arthritis, polyarteritis nodosa. Recovery from acute infections. *Skin diseases:* Psoriasis, pemphigus *Cancers:* Hodgkin's disease, eosinophilic leukemia	Typhoid fever, aplastic anemia and adrenal steroids
Basophils (<1% 0–100/cumm)	Chronic myeloid leukemia, polycythemia vera, myxedema, following splenectomy, Hodgkin's disease, urticaria pigmentosa, chickenpox, tuberculosis, influenza, smallpox	After administration of glucocorticoids Drug induced reactions
Lymphocytes (20–45% 1500–4000/cumm)	*Absolute:* Tuberculosis, brucellosis, syphilis, mumps, rubella, infectious mononeucleosis, leukemia and thyrotoxicosis *Relative:* All causes of neutropenia, infective hepatitis, convalescence from acute infections, infants with infections, malnutrition and avitaminosis	Severe bone marrow failure Immunosuppressive therapy Hodgkin's disease Irradiation AIDS
Monocytes (2–8% 200–800/cumm)	Chronic bacterial infections, protozoan diseases, Hodgkin's disease, chronic neutropenia, monocytic leukemia, rheumatic diseases	Aplastic anemia or hypoplastic bone marrow

Absolute Eosinophil Count

The normal range varies from 40 to 400 cells/cumm of blood.

Determination of Reticulocyte Count

The normal range in infants varies from 0.8 to 4% and in adults it varies from 0.8 to 2.5%. Increase in the count, i.e. reticulocytosis may be observed at birth, during pregnancy and menstruation. Pathological increase is seen in conditions such as, hemolytic anemia, pernicious anemia and sickle cell anemia. Decreased count is seen in aplastic anemia, myelofibrosis, radiation sickness and cytotoxic drug therapy.

Determination of Platelet Count

Platelets are the smallest blood cells, with the normal count of 1.5–4 lac/cumm. With recent technologic advances, accurate platelet counts are now widely available as a component of automated blood counts. The counts are done in a few seconds using either an electronic particle counting method (e.g. Coulter S-plus) or an optical method (e.g. Ortho ELT 8). An increased count i.e. thrombocytosis is observed in polycythemia vera, after administration of epinephrine due to splenic contraction, acute rheumatic fever, stress or after trauma (surgery, injury, child birth), in hemolytic anemia, disseminated intravascular coagulation, myeloproliferative disorders (particularly myelofibrosis), the Bernard–Soulier syndrome, and the May–Heggelin anomaly.

Thrombocytopenia or a decreased count is observed in bone marrow depression secondary to irradiation or drug hypersensitivity, hypersplenism, viral infection, acute and chronic leukemia, megaloblastic and aplastic anemia and subacute bacterial endocarditis.

Determination of Bleeding Time

When a small slit is made in the skin, the hemostatic mechanisms necessary for coagulation are activated. Without the aid of external pressure, bleeding usually stops within 7 to 9 minutes. Bleeding time (BT) measures the time taken from the start of the bleeding to until the bleeding stops. Bleeding time is said to be prolonged when bleeding time is more than 15 minutes. It can be measured using 2 methods: Duke's method (normal value—1–5 minutes) and Ivy's method (normal value—2–8 minutes).

Increased bleeding time is observed in thrombocytopenia, patients under aspirin therapy and those with Von Willebrand's disease and dissemination intravascular coagulation.

Determination of Clotting Time

There are 3 methods to measure clotting time, capillary tube method, Lee and White method and Kruse and Moses method. The normal clotting time (CT) according to these methods are 1–7 minutes, 5–10 minutes and 2.5–5 minutes respectively. Variations in the normal range are reported in Hemophilia, Von Willebrand's disease, a fibrinogenemia and dysfibrinogenemia.

Determination of Clot Retraction Time

Clot retraction qualitatively begins at 1–6 hours and completes within 24 hours and quantitatively 80–89% of the clot retracts within this time. Clot lysis time is within 72 hours. Clot retraction time is affected by: deficiency of platelets, poor platelet function, decreased fibrinogen, anemia, polycythemia and hyperglobinemia.

Determination of Prothrombin Time

The prothrombin time (PT) measures the time necessary to generate fibrin after activation of factor VII. It measures the integrity of the 'extrinsic' and 'common' pathways (factors VII, V, X, prothrombin, and fibrinogen). Prothrombin time is now commonly reported with INR (International normalized ratio), which is the ratio of prothrombin time that adjusts for the sensitivity of the thromboplastin reagents, such that a normal coagulation profile is reported as an INR of 1.0. The INR was introduced by WHO in 1983. The normal prothrombin time is estimated to be 10–15 seconds according to Quick's one stage method. Prothrombin time is prolonged in the following cases:

- Therapy with coumarin
- Heparin therapy
- Obstructive jaundice
- Liver disease
- Congenital deficiency of clotting factors II, V, VII, X
- Fibrinogen deficiency
- Vitamin K deficiency
- Hemorrhagic disease of newborn.

Determination of Partial Thromboplastin Time

It varies from 30–50 seconds. It is prolonged in the following cases:

- Anticoagulant therapy
- Hemophilia A
- Christmas disease
- Von Willebrand's disease
- Hepatic failure
- Factor II, V, X, XI or XII deficiency
- Disseminated intravascular coagulation
- Systemic lupus erythematosis.

Determination of Activated Partial Thromboplastin Time

Activated partial thromboplastin time (aPTT) is used to evaluate the intrinsic cascade and measure the functional levels of factors VIII, IX, XI and XII. It is a good screening test for inherited or acquired factor deficiencies. It is altered in inherited disorders such as hemophilia A and B and rarely in the absence of other intrinsic and common pathway factors. Acquired factor deficiency is common. Vitamin K deficiency, liver dysfunction, and iatrogenic anticoagulation with warfarin are most common. The normal aPTT time is 15–35 seconds.

Determination of Thrombin Time

Thrombin time (TT) is used to test the ability to form initial clot from fibrinogen. It measures the integrity of this reaction and isolates an abnormality to either a decrease in normal fibrinogen or an inhibitor to its activation. It normally is <20 seconds. Thrombin time is prolonged in the following cases:

- Heparin, fibrinogen or fibrin degradation products
- Hypofibrinogenemia
- Dysfibrinogenemia
- Chronic liver disease
- Multiple myeloma
- Disseminated intravascular coagulation.

Capillary Fragility Test or Tourniquet Test

Capillary fragility test indicates the degree of permeability of the capillary walls and any defect in them. Normally, petechiae in men do not exceed 5, and in women and children they do not exceed 10 per 1 inch circle.

Bone Marrow Aspiration

It is used in evaluation of patients with anemia, leukemia, metastatic malignancy and multiple myeloma.

A bone marrow biopsy is used when an indication of spatial relationship and degree of hyperplasia and hypoplasia of cellular elements in marrow is needed. The specimen is obtained from crest of ileum and the histologic sections are stained with Wright's stain.

Sickle Cell Preparation

Sickle cell preparation can be demonstrated *in vitro* by observing the cells in drop of blood diluted with sodium bisulfate and sealed on microscopic slide. In a positive test elongated, curved cells with multiple pointed extrusions are revealed after 10–15 minutes.

Hemoglobin Electrophoresis

The presence and relative concentration of various types of hemoglobin in various hemoglobinopathies are measured more accurately by electrophoresis of hemoglobin contained in red blood cells. In sickle cell disease 75–95% of hemoglobin on electrophoresis is found to be abnormal HbS and remainder fetal HbF. In sickle cell trait 20–45% of hemoglobin is HbS and remainder adult HbA.

Schilling's Test

It is indicated in pernicious anemia. The Schilling test is used to determine whether the body absorbs vitamin B_{12} normally.

Serum Iron and Total Iron Binding Capacity

Serum iron is the amount of iron bound to transferring in the plasma. It ranges from 55 to 185 μgm/cumm. The total iron binding capacity is the total amount of iron that can be bound to plasma transferring. The normal value ranges from 250 to 425 μgm/cumm.

Increased serum iron level is observed in hemolytic anemia, lead poisoning, pyridoxine deficiency and necrotic hepatitis, while total iron binding capacity increases in chronic blood loss and nephrosis. The total iron binding capacity decreases in cases with cirrhosis, hemochromatosis and nephrosis.

Serum Fibrinogen

The normal range varies from 200 to 400 mg/dL.

Estimation of Blood Sugar

Sugar particularly glucose, are the metabolites of carbohydrate foods, which comes to blood as fuel and supply energy for cells. Sugar level in the blood is controlled by factors like metabolic, hormonal and renal mechanism. The 2 hormones, insulin and glucagon that primarily regulate the sugar level in the body are secreted by the α- and β-cells of the liver. Glucagon is responsible for hyperglycemia, while insulin helps in the entry and utilization of glucose by cells. Other hormones like adrenaline, thyroxine, corticosteroid, etc., also influence blood sugar level. Normal blood sugar level is estimated to be 80–110 mg/100 mL. Patients with a borderline value of 126 mg/dL are considered to be suspected patients of diabetes. Whereas, the fasting level of >126 mg/dL is diagnostic of diabetes. In coma patients the level may reach up to 800–1,000 mg/dL.

Office screening procedures such as Urinary test taper, dextrostix, visidex, chemstrip bG provide only a range of glucose concentration rather than the exact figure. Hence, the facilities of a laboratory are needed for more accurate measurement. The concentration of glucose is highest in the arterial circulation. Laboratory determinations are usually done on venous samples. If the venous circulation is delayed, such as by leaving a tourniquet on for a prolonged period of time, the concentration falls even further. Thus, samples should be obtained after releasing the tourniquet. Dentists may carry out elective periodontal and oral surgery procedures in diabetics only when the patient is under good metabolic control, for which an accurate blood glucose concentration is often needed. Detection of diabetes mellitus in dental patients is important owing to the following facts:

- The response of diabetic patient to periodontal therapy may be much less satisfactory than nondiabetic under similar conditions.
- The healing of oral tissues following surgery in the diabetic may be slower and may be subjected to more complication such as tissue necrosis and risk for a secondary infection.
- The systemic effects of acute localized oral infections may be much greater in diabetics than in the nondiabetic patients.
- Certain oral diseases are predisposed to occur in association with DM (e.g. thrush, denture sore mouth).
- It is a disease of insidious onset, which may range from serious tissue changes to permanent cardiovascular, renal, optic and cerebral damage.

Screening

Identifying and screening the affected individuals is based on the appropriate recording of the history of the patient along with the signs and symptoms of diabetes viz., polyuria, polydyspsia and polyphagia. Glucosuria is the testing of the urine with commercially available reagent strip such as, Tes tape, Clinistix, Chemstip. However, sometimes a false positive result may be observed in cases of:

- Renal glucosuria, which is a familial condition, characterized by a low renal threshold for glucose and normal blood glucose levels.
- Presence of other reducing sugars such as lactose in urine.
- If specific glucose oxidase containing reagent strip is not used for the process.

In confirmed cases with diabetes mellitus (DM), there are three schedules for determination of blood glucose:

1. *Fasting blood sugar:* It is used as a screening test for hyperglycemia in hospitalized patients. The normal value ranges from 80–110 mg/dL.

2. *Postprandial blood glucose:* It is a more sensitive measurement of the hyperglycemia associated with DM. Both fasting and postprandial blood glucose measurements can be carried out with capillary blood using the dextrostix, visidex or chemstrip bG+ reagents strips. Visidex and chemstrip bG strips are especially manufactured for visual color matching for accurate use. Dextrostix must be read with colorimeter. The special equipment available for the purpose is dextrometer in laboratory and in home glucometer reflectance photometer (GRP). A new GRP known as Accu-chek bG is available for patients who are unable to read chemstrip bG accurately from a color chart. Because of its convenience, simplicity and sensitivity it is the best screening procedure for dentist. The patient is asked to ingest approximately 75–100 g carbohydrate 2 hours prior the test. Urine also checked for glucose. Urine analysis is done using the Tes tape, clinistrix, chemstrip, diastix. It is indicated for:

- Evaluation in a patient suspected for having DM. Proper history should to be taken regarding weight loss, polyphagia, polydypsia, polyurea, any history of repeated boils, skin infections, and persistent infections and presence of similar condition in the family.
- As a screening test of diabetes for every patient over 50 years of age, patients with obesity and patient with relevant family history.
- As a measure of the degree of control of the disease in known diabetic patient.

The blood sugar concentration rises to about 160 mg/dL following meal but returns to normal level within 2 hours. In diabetic fasting level may reach 200 mg/dL and postprandial level are greater than this and may persist for longer than 2 hours after meal. Dextrostix, viridex and chemstrip bG estimates blood glucose concentration between the range of 40–250 mg/dL. Beyond this range reagent, strips tend to under estimate blood glucose concentration to a varying degree.

This test does usually differentiate between hyperglycemia and hypoglycemia and is useful in gross approximation of blood glucose control for diabetic outpatient. Urine is also checked for glucose. When blood sugar exceeds 160–180 mg/dL the glucose appears in urine. Urine analysis is done using the Tes tape, clinistrix, chemstrip, diastix. False negative result is seen in renal diseases. Glucosuria with hyperglycemia is caused by DM, hyperthyroidism, general anesthesia and intracranial lesions such as stroke. Whereas, glucosuria without hyperglycemia is seen in patients with renal glucosuria in 10–15% normal pregnancies, under stress and following ingestion of high carbohydrate meal. A false negative test may also be reported when glucose peroxidase is present with other reducing metabolites in the urine. Example: Patient consuming 2.4 g or more of aspirin daily, levodopa for Parkinson's syndrome or a patient with carcinoid syndrome. A false positive result may be anticipated if jars are contaminated with chlorhexidine antiseptic.

3. *Glucose tolerance test (GTT):* This test is used for the definitive diagnosis of DM. It is performed on a series of sample of blood and urine in patients who do not exhibit consistently elevated fasting sugar levels. It has been accepted as a procedure for making definitive diagnosis of DM and for distinguishing DM from other causes of hyperglycemia like hyperthyroidism. This test is advised when the patient's fasting plasma glucose is not elevated on more than one occasion. GTT is however, not necessary for known hyperglycemic patients. In such cases fasting and postprandial blood sugar estimation is sufficient. It is helpful in recognizing mild cases of diabetes and in identifying patients with symptom less glycosuria. GTT has little value in the following the course of treatment in diabetics.

Glucose tolerance means the ability of the body to utilize the glucose circulating in the blood. In normal individual blood glucose level remains constant throughout, whereas it is decreased in diabetics. Following ingestion of food, there is a temporary rise in blood sugar, the extent and duration of which depends on the type of food taken. This returns to the normal fasting level within 2–3 hours after the intake of food. This effect of ingested carbohydrate can be studied under standard conditions by means of glucose tolerance test. The procedure, however, takes longer time of about 3–5 hours and is also expensive when compared to the regular methods used in the estimation of blood sugar.

The patient is given 75 g of glucose or 50–100 g (1.75 g/kg wt) dissolved in water. Lemon juice may be added to avoid vomiting. The time is noted and 4 more samples within 2 hours, with an interval of half an hour are collected. 4 urine samples are also collected simultaneously after every blood sample (at least two urine samples at 1 hour interval). The blood and urine sugar is determined and a G tolerance curve is prepared by plotting time on x-axis and plasma glucose van on y-axis. The result is evaluated as follows:

- *Normal response:* The type of normal curve varies with age. In older patients maximum blood glucose level may be up to 170 mg/dL.
- *Diminished glucose tolerance:* This happens when ability of body to utilize glucose decreases, as is seen in DM.

- In glucose tolerance curve (GTC) 3 and 4 the rise in blood glucose is greater than the normal and the return of blood glucose to normal fasting level is delayed. GTC 3 shows mild diabetics with 1–2% sugar in urine. A similar curve can also be seen in:
  - Hyperactivity of the thyroid, adrenal and pituitary glands
  - Injection of ACTH or cortisone like hormone
  - Increased secretion of growth hormone
  - Severe liver disease (due to reduction in glycogen formation)
  - Glycogen storage diseases
  - Severe infection.

GTC 4 indicate severe diabetics with >2% urine sugar. GTC 2 is lag type of GTC (prediabetic). It is seen due to the temporary rise in blood sugar after ingestion of glucose as a result of delay in the insulin mechanism for coming into action. Blood glucose returns to normal limits in the usual time. But the peak of the curve is above the normal renal threshold. So there is transient glucosuria. GTC 5 indicates increased glucose tolerance, which is the ability of body to utilize more glucose. It is observed in cases of endocrine hypoactivity, such as hypothyroidism, hypoadrenalism (Addison's disease) and hypopituitarism. In certain conditions like idiopathic steatorrhea, celiac disease and sprue, the fasting blood sugar levels may sometimes be below the normal limits or only a small rise is observed in blood glucose.

Few important and relevant observations and the associated conditions are mentioned as under:

- *Raised renal threshold:* It is observed with increasing age and in patients with prolonged DM. The blood glucose level rises up to 250 mg/dL or more producing glucosuria.
- *Lower renal threshold:* It is seen in transient glucosuria due to the abnormality in tubular reabsorption of glucose.
- *Extended GTC for up to 2½ hours–5 hours:* If glucose level drops below 60 mg/dL after every 30 minutes, it may be due to insulin secreting tumors of pancreas, Simmond's disease.

Impaired glucose tolerance (IGT) is used to describe patient who fail to satisfy the criteria for diabetes but who fulfill the following three criteria:

1. Fasting blood glucose concentration must be below the value that is diagnostic of diabetes.
2. The glucose concentration 2 hours after 75 g oral glucose challenge must be between normal and diabetic values.
3. The value obtained 1/2, 1 or 1½ hours after test dose must be unequivocally elevated.

Glucose values above the normal concentration but below the criteria for diabetes or IGT should be considered nondiagnostic for either diabetes or IGT.

Glycosylated Hemoglobin

If a patient is known to have diabetes, it is critical that the level of glycemic control be established before initiating the treatment. The fasting glucose and casual glucose tests provide snapshots of the blood glucose concentration at the time the blood was drawn; these tests reveal nothing about long-term glycemic control in a known diabetic individual is the glycosylated (or glycated) hemoglobin (Hb) assay.

The red cells of normal human adults and children above 6 months of age contain 3 Hb species: HbA (90%), HbA_2 (2.5%) and HbF (0.5%). Beside these Hb other variants, the products of nonenzymatic, postsynthetic transformation of HbA are also present: HbA_{1a} (1.6%), HbA_{1b} (0.8%) and HbA_{1c} (4.0%). Glycosylated Hb is normally formed in circulating blood by nonenzymatic addition of hexose molecules to N-terminal valine of the β-chains of HbA. The more commonly measured glycosylated Hb is HbA_{1c} that contain one or 2 molecule of glucose attached to each HbA molecules. The percentage of hemoglobin glycosylated depends on the average glucose concentration the red cell is exposed to over time. Since the average life of the red cell is 120 days, the HbA_{1c} assay gives a good indication of the degree of blood sugar control over the preceding 6–8 weeks and may provide an indication of the potential response to dental therapy.

Various methods for the estimation of glycosylated Hb are:

- Spectrophotometric colorimeter
- Ion exchange method
- Isoelectric focusing
- Radioimmunoassay

Patients with relatively well-controlled diabetes (HbA_{1c} <8%) usually respond to treatment in a manner similar to nondiabetics. Poorly controlled patients (HbA_{1c} >10%) often have a poor response to treatment, with more postoperative complications and less favorable long-term results. Certain conditions, such as uremia, aspirin ingestion, and alcoholism, can cause spurious elevations of glycosylated hemoglobin. Falsely low percentages of glycosylate Hb can be caused by uremia, anemia, variant hemoglobins such as hemoglobin S, and pregnancy. The sensitivity of the measurement of hemoglobin A_{1c} is such that the test cannot be used to diagnose diabetes, but it is a useful means of following the blood glucose control of the diabetic patient.

Urine Blood Sugar

It is measured by titration. When glucose is mixed with Benedict's reagent, it reduces cupric ions in the solution to cuprous ions on reacting with potassium thiocyanate to form white colored cuprous thiocyanate. As precipitate formed is white, the loss of all blue color indicates complete reduction of cupric ions.

Microbiological Investigations

The association of microbial agents with oral disease may be demonstrated either by recognizing characteristic microorganisms in smears prepared from the lesions, by preparing a culture of the isolated agent, by measuring the concentration of specific antibodies to the microorganism in serum or saliva or by recognizing characteristic tissue changes or microorganisms in biopsies. These are beneficial in:

- Isolation and identification of causative organism from the pathological lesions and to find the source of infection.
- Prognosis of the disease.
- Guidance in treatment by culturing the organism and then performing drug sensitivity test.

The normal bacterial flora of the body consists of symbionts, commensals and opportunistic microorganisms. The range of the organisms depends on patient's age, sex, race, nutrition, environment and hormonal activity. The common microorganisms found in the oral cavity are enterobacteriae, *Neisseria sp., Lactobacillus sp., Corneybacterium sp., Staphylococcus aureus, Staphylococcus epidermis* and *Haemophilus sp.*

Isolation of the Oral Microbial Flora

Oral cavity possess extremely high microbial flora. Most of the infectious oral diseases are mixed endogenous infections derived from microbial flora; therefore bacterial isolation has limited value in oral disease diagnosis. But it is indicated in certain suppurative lesions, where it also aid in diagnosis and to identify the pathogens and treatment planning. Identification of the organisms present in the pus aspirated from the lesions can provide information on the nature of the infection. The lesion which fails to respond to the initial antibiotic therapy should be subjected to isolation and antibiotic sensitivity test. If pus or the specimen is contaminated with saliva the more rapidly growing members will appear on the inoculated medium. Sometime cultures inoculated with aspirated pus will fail to grow. This indicates sterility of the pus or the presence of any organism likely to grow on the media used.

Specimen Collection and Procedure

The specimen should be collected with the help of a swab under ascetic technique. The specimen is inoculated directly or taken to the laboratory immediately. If a delay is expected put the specimen in transport medium. A single bacteriologic medium or culture technique does not allow the isolation of all the microorganisms. Therefore, when a particular organism is suspected to be the cause it should be informed to the laboratory; which makes it easier for the laboratory to use the specific culture. The common culture medias used in dentistry are:

- *Blood agar media:* For streptococci differentiates (α, β and γ *Streptococcus*)
- Lowestein-Jensen media for *Mycobacterium* tuberculosis and Bovine.
- Robertstein's cooked meat media for anaerobic microbes.
- Sugar media or carbohydrate fermentation media with serum peptone water for *Neisseria* and *Corynebacterium.*
- Mcleod's blood tellurite media for *Corynebacterium.*

Transient bacteremia can be demonstrated in 70–90% patients during extraction and periodontal surgery. It may lead to bacterial endocarditis in rheumatic valvulitis patients with rheumatic valvulitis, patients with congenital heart disease or who have undergone a cardiac surgery. Bacterial endocarditis may also occur as a complication of the infectious process and surgical manipulation elsewhere in the body. The persistent bacteremia in endocarditis patients may be detected by inoculating 5–10 mL of venous blood into appropriate culture media. Positive blood culture indicates septicemia or bacterial endocarditis. Bacteremia may not be continuously present, hence repeated tests over several days may be done before a positive culture is obtained.

Cultures of Tooth Apices

Cultures made from the apical region of extracted teeth by various techniques must be interpreted very carefully as they may be contaminated with oral microbial flora. An external approach or a root amputation method of culturing is preferable. The patients do not easily agree for this method as it requires additional surgical procedures. The most preferred teeth are the maxillary anterior teeth with single root. It is difficult to render the sterility of the operative field, particularly with gingival sulcular fluid. The most effective method of sterilizing gingival sulcus is cauterization by heat before extraction of teeth.

Bacterial Cultures in Endodontics

Most commonly gram-positive organisms (75%) are found in the root canals, but gram-negative and obligate anaerobes (25%) have also been found in the root canals. Usually, the microorganisms which can survive in environment of low oxygen tension and can survive the rigors of limited pabulums are found in the root canals. Variety of microorganisms enters the root canals through various portals of entry such as, open cavity, open dentinal tubules, faulty restorations, anachoresis and periodontal ligament or gingival sulcus, but only those whish are fit to survival in such environment do survive. These microorganisms can be detected with the help of gram staining or culturing of the root canals. Root canal cultures are indicated for:

- Endodontic treatment of nonvital teeth.
- Teeth with persistent pain and discomfort
- Teeth that present with exudates in canal or an area of periapical pathosis.
- Apical infectious process requiring careful selection of antibiotics.

For culturing samples may be obtained from either from an infected root canal or from a periradicular abscess. Various media used as culturing material are as follows:

- Brain heart infusion broth with 0.1% agar.
- Trypticase soy broth 0.1% agar for anaerobic organisms.
- 10% horse serum.
- Thioglycollate.
- Glucose ascites broth for fastidious organisms.

Sometimes negative culture becomes positive after 24–48 hours. Hence, it is advised to allow more than 48 hours between taking culture and obturation of the root canal.

Examination of Microbial Flora from Plaque and Gingival Crevice

Scraping from dental plaque and gingival crevice are used for educating the patients regarding effectiveness of home care procedures and in research lab and periodontal office to estimate the proportions of the subgingival spirochetes and motile bacteria as a predictor of containing periodontal destruction.

Deep pockets show the presence of spirochetes without motile bacteria. Dark field microscope examination in patients with progressive periodontitis has shown an average of 16–28% of spirochetes and motile rods in the crevice flora. 2–7% microorganisms were found in cases where periodontal destruction was halted. Subgingival microbial flora estimation has predictive value in determining effectiveness of home care procedure and in professional procedures like curettage and prophylactic procedure. They aid in prognosis of individual periodontal involved teeth and need for surgical treatment.

Caries Activity Tests

Clinical examination of carious lesions with probe and mirror, coupled with radiographs, neither predicts caries nor a patient's susceptibility to caries. A reliable laboratory test for measuring caries activity offers a valuable adjunct for patient motivation in a caries prevention program. Caries activity refers to the increment of active lesions (new and recurrent lesions) over a stipulated period of time. These tests identify the individual with high cariogenic potential and measure the degrees to which local environmental challenge favors the probability of carious lesions. Whereas, caries susceptibility refers to the inherent tendency of the host and target tissue, the tooth to be afflicted by the carious process. These tests help determine the need for personalized preventive measures, motivation for the patient, monitor the effectiveness of oral health education programs and serve as an index of the success of therapeutic measures by monitoring patient behavior towards reducing the number of *S. mutans* and lactobacilli as part of counseling to reduce sucrose intake.

Several biochemical and microbiological tests which are suitable for use in dental clinics and offices have been developed as indices for caries activity as illustrated below.

Lactobacillus Colony Count Test

It is the oldest and widely used test for assessing caries activity, which was proposed by Hadley in 1933. It measures the number of aciduric bacteria in the patient's saliva by counting the number of colonies that appear on tomato peptone agar plates, a selective medium with pH 5.0, after inoculation of patient's saliva and incubation. 5 mL of stimulated saliva is collected in a sterile container and shaken for 2 minutes. Saliva is diluted to 1:10 with distilled water. It is again diluted to 1:100 and mixed thoroughly. This sample is spread on the surface of agar plates and inoculated for 3–4 days at 37° C. the lactobacilli count is interpreted as follows:

Number of lactobacilli/mL	*Degree of caries activity*
0–1000	Little or no activity
1000–5000	Slight activity
5000–10.000	Moderate activity
>10,000	Marked activity

Colorimetric Synder Test

This test was developed by Synder in 1951. It measures the ability of salivary microorganisms to form organic acids from a carbohydrate medium. The medium has a color indicator such as bromocresol green, which changes from blue-green at pH 4.7–5.0 to yellow at pH 4.0. Incubation of saliva and it is mixed with bromocresol green dextrose agar at 37°C and pH 5.0. the acid produced is detected by the changes in pH indicator, and is compared to an uninoculated control tube after 24, 48 and 72 hours. The test estimates the number of both acidogenic and aciduric bacteria. The color observations are as follows:

Time (in hours)	*24*	*48*	*72*
Color	Yellow	Yellow	Yellow
Caries activity	Marked	Definite	Limited
Color	Green	Green	Green
Caries activity	Test to be continued	Test to be continued	Inactive

Swab Test

This test was developed by Grainger et al. in 1965. No collection of saliva is necessary unlike other tests and hence is valuable in evaluating caries activity in very young children. The test involves sampling of the oral flora by swabbing buccal surfaces of teeth with cotton swab and incubating it in the medium. The pH change is read on a pH meter after 48 hours of incubation and interpreted as follows:

pH	*Caries activity*
≤4	Marked activity
4.2–4.4	Active
4.5–4.6	Slightly active
>4.6	Caries inactive

Salivary *S. mutans* Level Test

The number of *S. mutans* forming units per unit volume of saliva is the basic principle of this test. Incubation of sample obtained using tongue blades or wooden spatula is done on Mitis Salivarius Agar (MSA) at 37°C for 48 hours 95% N_2-5% CO_2. This test does not differentiate caries and cariogenic state and *S. mutans* tends to be located at specific sites only. Levels of *S. mutans* >10^5 CFU/mL are indicative of unacceptable cariogenic challenge, since colonization does not occur until the level of *S. mutans* reaches 4.5×10^4 CFU/mL for smooth surface caries and 10^3 CFU/mL for occlusal fissures.

S. mutans Dip Slide Method

This test classifies salivary samples according to estimates of *S. mutans* colonies growing on modified MSA. A zone of inhibition is formed around each bacitracin disc. If present, these organisms appear as small blue colonies growing within the zone of inhibition. The colony density is classified as 0 (negligible), 1 (<1,00,000 CFU/mL), 2 (1,00,000-10,00,000 CFU/mL) and 3 (>10,00,000 CFU/ mL).

Salivary Buffer Capacity Test

This test measures the quantity of acid required to lower the pH of saliva through an arbitrary pH interval. It relates the buffering capacity of saliva and caries activity. Patients with increased susceptibility to dental caries show a lower buffering capacity in their saliva than saliva of patients who are caries free.

Enamel Solubility Test

It is also known as the Fosdick calcium dissolution test. It measures the milligrams of powdered enamel dissolved in 4 hours by acid formed when the patient's saliva is mixed with glucose and powdered enamel. The test, however, is not simple and expensive, yet in limited studies, the correlation reported is good. This test is not suitable for office procedures.

Salivary Reductase Test

This test measures the rate at which the indicator molecules diazoresorcinol, changes from blue to red to colorless or whitish on reduction by the mixed salivary flora. The test measures the activity of salivary reductase enzyme present in the salivary bacteria. It requires no incubation process and caries conduciveness reading is taken in 15 minutes and interpreted as follows:

Time	*Color*	*Score*	*Caries activity*
15 minutes	Blue	1	Nonconductive
15 minutes	Orchid	2	Slightly conducive
15 minutes	Red	3	Moderately conducive
Immediately	Red	4	Highly conducive
Immediately	Pink/White	5	Extremely conducive

Other Tests

Alban Test

It is a simplified substitute for the Synder test. It uses a simpler sampling procedure where the patient expectorates directly into tubes that contain the medium.

Streptococcus Mutans Screening Test

It can be done by 2 methods namely plaque/tooth pick method and saliva/tongue blade method. The plaque method involves a simple screening of diluted plaque sample streaked on a selective culture media. It is an attempt to semiquantitatively screen the dental plaque for a specific group of caries inducing *S. mutans*. The tongue blade method was developed for use in large number of school children. It estimates the number of *S. mutans* in mixed paraffin stimulated saliva when cultured on Mutans Salivarius Bacitracin Agar.

Ora Test

The test developed by Rosenberg et al. in 1989 is based on the rate of oxygen depletion by microorganisms in expectorated milk samples. It is used for estimating oral microbial levels.

Biopsy

Biopsy is defined as the removal of tissue from the living organisms for the purpose of microscopic examination and diagnosis. It is one of the most valuable supplementary diagnostic aids and is used to confirm a presumptive diagnosis made on clinical and radiographic findings. Biopsy is the gold standard diagnostic procedure to obtain adequate representative tissue for histopathological evaluation to arrive at final diagnosis. The various types of biopsy techniques are:

- Needle biopsy
- Punch biopsy
- Brush biopsy
- *Open biopsy:* Further divided as incisional and excisional.

A biopsy is indicated in the following cases:

- Any ulcer that has not shown evidence of healing in 21 days.
- Any tumor that is suspected of being neoplastic.
- Any persistent hyperkeratotic lesion.
- Any intraosseous lesion that cannot be positively identified radiographically.
- Any tissue that has been surgically removed or spontaneously expelled from a body orifice.
- Material from persistent draining sinus.

Few things should be kept in mind when doing a biopsy:

- Specimen should be removed with a minimum of manipulation of area.

- Pigmented lesion should be excised with wide margin of the normal tissue surrounding the lesion.
- In case of small lesion entire lesion acts, as specimen and it should be removed completely. Whereas, in large lesion specimen is moved from most easily accessible area.
- Thin deep sections are more desirable than large shallow specimen.
- If several lesions are present the specimen should be taken from the most representative.
- Lesions that are vascular in origin should be removed in initial procedure as it may result in extensive hemorrhage.
- If the lesion is intraosseous the cortical plate of bone should be removed along with margin.
- Local anesthesia should never be injected into the lesion.
- Time between the taking of the specimen and reporting the diagnosis should be as short as possible.

Procedure

- Tissue should be removed with sharp instrument and with minimum manipulation.
- Specimen should be immediately placed in a fixative and should not be left in air to dry.
- The container should have a wide mouth to permit the specimen to be dropped in fixative and have leak proof capsule. 10% formalin is commonly used as fixative, but other special fixatives are also used.
- If there are more than one specimen then each should placed in different containers.
- Patients' age, name, sex, and any other information regarding lesion should be attached to outside the container.
- Specimen should be sent or mailed to the pathology laboratory immediately.

Fine Needle Aspiration Biopsy

Aspiration is a means of obtaining material from body cavity, cystic space, or a fluid containing lesion. In fine needle aspiration biopsy (FNAB), the doctor uses a very thin needle attached to a syringe to aspirate a small amount of tissue from the suspicious area. This tissue is then looked at under a microscope. The needle used for FNAB is thinner than the ones that are used for blood tests. Examples of various types of needles that are used for various masses:

- *For bony lesions:* 18 gauze
- *Neck, Thyroid, Breast masses:* 18–20 gauze
- *Neck masses:* 21 gauze
- *Salivary gland tumors:* 25 or 23 gauze.

The technique is used for palpable masses such as: enlarged lymph nodes, bony lesions, salivary glands, enlarged thyroid, breast masses, superficial soft tissue masses and palpable abdominal lesions.

Procedure

After putting the patient in supine position, locate and palpate the lesion and give anesthesia. Pass the needle through the skin and advance the needle into lesion. Apply suction and move the needle repeatedly through mass in various directions. Release suction. Remove the needle from patient. Detach the needle from syringe. Fill syringe with air. Replace the needle onto syringe and change grip on syringe holder. Touch the needle tip to a microscope slide to express the specimen onto the slide. Prepare the smear. Fix or dry the smear.

Advantages

- It is a simple technique with greater patient acceptance.
- It is a safe and reliable method of diagnosing suspected lesions in the head and neck region.
- There is less risk of delayed wound healing and infection.
- It eliminates the need for hospitalization and saves the operating room time.
- The risk of seeding the needle track with cancer cells that accompanies the use of a large needle is unlikely with FNAB.
- Different areas within the mass can be easily sampled.
- It is a definitive diagnostic technique and allows the clinician to begin the treatment.

Various colored aspirated material obtained from various lesions:

Color of the aspirated material	*Lesion*
Straw color	Odontogenic cyst, cystic ameloblastoma
Firm, viscous aspirate	Epidermoid cyst
Yellowish to gray, i.e. Sebum	Sebaceous cyst
Thickest yellowish cheesy substance	Dermoid cyst
Thick yellowish white granular fluid	Lumina of epithelial cyst, keratocyst
Dark amber colored fluid	Thyroglossal duct cyst
Bluish blood	Early hematomas, hemangiomas, varicosities
Bright red cooler	Aneurysm, AV shunt
Yellowish white pus with sulfur granules	Actinomycosis
Cloudy and frothy colorless fluid	Lymphangioma, cystic hygroma
Sticky, clear viscous fluid	Retention phenomenon, tumor of minor salivary gland
Yellow to yellowish white	Odontogenic infection
Thin straw colored fluid	Papillary cystic adenoma, papillary cystadenoma lymphomatosum
Soft masses filled with air	Subcutaneous emphysema, laryngoceles
Mucous aspiration	Low grade mucoepidermoid carcinoma

Exfoliative Cytology

Exfoliative cytology is the microscopic examination of cells which exfoliate or abrade from the body surfaces. When the epithelium becomes the seat of any pathological condition, the cells may lose their cohesiveness and cells in the deeper layer may shed along with the superficial cells. These cells by means of specific instruments can be studied quantitatively and qualitatively. Application of cytodiagnosis as a routine procedure in the detection of cervical cancer was introduced by Dr George N Papanicolaou in 1941. Oral exfoliative cytology was introduced by Silvermann and Sandler.

Indications

It has been recognized that oral exfoliative cytology is of value in the diagnosis of diseases other than carcinoma, particularly diseases which are characterized by the presence of certain specific cells. Thus it is useful in the diagnosis of herpes simplex infection, herpes zoster, pemphigus vulgaris, white sponge nevus, hereditary benign intraepithelial dyskeratosis, keratosis follicularis, benign familial pemphigus and pernicious and sickle cell anemia. It is indicated when the lesion is question is so innocuous as not to arouse suspicion of cancer and when the lesion is located in inaccessible areas. When there is resistance on the part of either the dentist or patient to have a biopsy performed then exfoliative cytology may be used to confirm the diagnosis. It is also indicated in cases when there are large multiple red lesions and best site for a biopsy cannot be determined. It is also recommended as a follow-up procedure for detection of recurrent cancer in previously treated patient.

Contraindications

An obvious or suspected cancer that would justify taking a biopsy specimen is not indicated for exfoliative cytology. It is also contraindicated for a patient who cannot be relied on to keeping a second appointment for follow-up examination of lesion. It is contraindicated for submucosal lesions, dry or crusted lesion as may be seen on the lips and white lesion that does not rub off.

Procedure

The procedure is a simple one, which consists essentially of cleansing the surface of the oral lesion of debris and mucin and then vigorously scraping the entire surface several times with a metal cement spatula, a moistened tongue blade or a cytobrush. If spatula is used the material is spread on one slide and another drawn across it. If cotton tipped applicator is used the material is smeared on both slides with an applicator. It is then immersed in fixative for 30 minutes, since the slightest air drying will cause distortion of cells and air dried. The fixative may be a commercial preparation such as Spray-cyte, 95% alcohol, or equal parts alcohol and ether. Slides are never flame fixed as bacteriologic smears. Slides are prepared for shipment together with clinical information available. This information should include name, address of the sender and of the patient, age, sex and race of patient, the duration and location of the lesion and its description. It is essential that the procedure be repeated and a second smear be prepared for submission to the cytologist. In the preparation of the second slide, a separate scraping should be utilized.

The cytologic smear will usually be reported by the cytologist as under one of the following classes:

Class I (Normal)	Only normal cells are present
Class II (Atypical)	Minor atypia present but no evidence of malignant changes
Class III (Intermediate)	The cells display wider atypia that may be suggestive of cancer, but they are not clear-cut and may represent precancerous lesions or carcinoma *in situ*. It separates cancer from noncancer diagnosis and biopsy is recommended
Class IV (Suggestive of cancer	A few cells with malignant characteristics or many cells with borderline characteristics. Biopsy is mandatory
Class V (Positive for cancer)	Cells that are obviously malignant and biopsy is mandatory

Advantages

Limited equipment is needed for this simple and inexpensive procedure. It can be done without anesthesia or surgical instruments. Less time is required than other methods. It does not cause anxiety or fear of cancer to patients.

Disadvantages

Though it has a significant role in diagnosis of cancer, it has its own limitations. It detects only surface lesions and the presence or extent of invasion cannot be assessed. If surface is keratinized then typical character of the lesion will not be demonstrated by the limited material. Treatment cannot be predicted on a positive smear; a biopsy is still necessary to verify the positive lesion. Exfoliative cells in the oral lesions are continually washed away. Negative report provides a false security of having adequately surveyed the area or lesion. A positive smear indicates the need for a biopsy; the negative smear means very little. Exfoliate cytology is inadequate as a screening procedure. Majority of benign lesions that occur in the oral cavity do not lend themselves to cytologic smears, e.g. fibroma and leukoplakia.

Punch Biopsy

Biopsy punches range in size from 2 to 6 mm in diameter. Depth of the biopsy punch used is 4 mm for most diseases. 3 mm and 6 mm punches are employed frequently. Biopsy punches are of the following types:

- *Keyes biopsy punch:* Size range from 1.0 to 12.0 mm in increments of 0.25–0.50 mm.

- *Belt driven punch:* It has a speed of 250–36,000 rpm and weighs 25 g.
- *Disposable biopsy punch:* It weighs 2 g and has a better access to different areas.

Punch biopsies are used as an incisional biopsy for the purpose of diagnosis, before definitive therapy, for mucosal neoplasm, reactive processes and when there are signs of mucocutaneous diseases.

Technique

After selecting the biopsy site; it is anesthetized and gently blotted with sterile gauze. The edge of the biopsy punch blade is placed on oral mucosa and rotated back and forth between the fingers until the external bevel is no longer visible. If adequate depth is not obtained then punch is withdrawn and the need for additional depth is assessed. If necessary, the punch can be replaced in the original position and procedure can be continued until appropriate depth is reached. The base of the tissue core is released by using No. 15 scalpel blade or fine curved iris scissors. Appropriate fixative such as, 10% neutral buffered formalin is used. Thereafter, the patient is given postoperative instructions.

Advantages

It has low incidence of postsurgical morbidity. Suturing is not required and hence there is minimal or no scar formation resulting in maximum esthetic results. There is no need for postoperative or suture removal visit. It can be used on any mucosal surface that is assessable to biopsy punch.

Disadvantages

- This technique is designed for use only with epithelial or superficial mesenchymal lesions.
- It should be used with caution when lesion over lie significant submucosal structures such as mental or nasopalatine foramina.
- Freely movable mucosa that cannot be well-supported as with floor of mouth and soft pallet may preclude the technique.
- Access to maxillary posterior buccal alveolar ridge and anterior lingual aspect of mandible is difficult.
- It is difficult to use when adequate representative tissue deeper than superficial lamina propria has to be obtained.

Brush Biopsy

Brush biopsy is a method of detecting oral precancerous and cancerous lesions. There is minimal or no bleeding in this rapidly conducted chair side procedure. No topical or local anesthesia is needed. Recent brush used for brush biopsy is Oral CDx brush. Color margins of abnormalities from Oral CDx images enable dentist to demonstrate to the patient the abnormal test result.

Procedure

Depending on the lesions intraoral location and accessibility either flat surface or circular border of brush is placed on surface of the lesion. Firm pressure is maintained and brush is rotated for 5–10 times. Pinkness of tissue or pinpoint bleeding at the brush biopsy site is evidence of proper technique. Cellular material collected on brush is transferred to bar-coded glass slide and rapidly flooded with fixative to avoid air drying. After 15 minutes the slide is placed in a plastic container and sent with bar coded requisition form, in the pre-addressed mailing container.

Oral CDx slide is stained with papanicolaou method. Stained slide is scanned with computer system. This does not provide diagnosis of brush biopsy specimen but assists in identification of abnormal cells, which are then visually assessed by pathologist who confirms the final diagnosis.

Artifact

An artifact refers to an artificial structure or tissue alteration on a prepared microscopic slide as the result of an extraneous factor. Artifacts are the integral part of each microscopic field. Sometimes they can create serious errors and misdiagnosis. Artifacts may arise as a result of faulty surgical technique or correspond to sample processing in the laboratory. Biopsies of the oral cavity are of small size and fine texture; as a result, artifacts are easily produced during processing, microtomy and staining procedures. These artifacts result in alteration of normal morphologic and cytological features or even complete uselessness of the tissue, interfering with providing a correct histopathological impression. It is important to identify the common occurring artifacts during interpretation of oral biopsies.

Types of Artifacts

- *Fragmentation and hemorrhage:* Excessive stretching of the tissue during biopsy procedure usually results in fragmentation of the specimen and may even produce hemorrhage at the margins or within the tissue.
- *Effects of fulguration and laser:* Necrosis at the margins of the biopsy specimen is observed in the samples which are biopsied or removed by electrocautery or CO_2 laser.
- *Effects of inadequate and excessive fixation:* Inadequate fixation resulted in loss of tissue architecture, formation of vacuoles; improper staining, etc. Distinction between different tissue components was also difficult in some samples due to fixation for insufficient duration.
- *Improper orientation:* If the specimen is too small, such as a delicate strip of oral mucosa, the shrinking process due to formalin fixation causes curling and bending of the tissue, making difficult the correct orientation during the embedding procedure. Evaluation of epithelium becomes extremely difficult when such alterations are present.

- *Processing and microtomy artifacts:* Most common artifacts corresponding to the tissue processing are observed due to improper fixation.
- *Artifacts due to improper handling of sections:* Horizontal and vertical splits were frequently produced when the cut sections were not handled properly.
- *Staining artifacts:* Pertaining to staining procedure, the most common artifact is improper differentiation, i.e. lack of contrast between basophilic and eosinophilic components of the tissues. Precipitations of the staining solution and impurities are noted when old staining solutions were used.
- *Artifacts due to improper cover sliding:* Air bubbles are frequently noted appearing as transparent glistening ring like structures between coverslide and the section. Inclusions of foreign material, tiny pieces of glass from the broken cover slide, fibers of cotton and dust particles are recognizable because they are in different plane from that of tissue section.
- *Contamination by air borne fungi:* Common air inhabitant fungi like *Alternaria* and *Leptothrix* contaminated the mounting medium in slides which are very old or in which old mounting medium is used.

Frozen Sections

These are used for the initial study to obtain histologic diagnosis when a definitive therapeutic procedure is to be carried out immediately. They are used for the assessment of adequacy of surgical excision by a check of margins of resection. These are also indicated for preliminary assessment of nature of planned procedure, as determined by extent and distribution of tissue involved by a tumor, for diagnosis of any abnormality of tissue observed during surgery and to determine if a lesion requires immediate or special handling.

Frozen sections are contraindicated if the tissue is heavily calcified or ossified or if the tissue specimen is small. It is also contraindicated for lesions that even under optimum conditions require extensive study because of their complexity such as, lymphoreticular disorders, small superficial lytic lesions and some granulomatous diseases.

Advantages

- Preserves tissue section morphology and integrity and localization of tissue sections.
- It eliminates the tears, precious material losses, tissue folds and compressions.
- It allows ultra thin sections down to 2 μm.
- It is ideal for reliable and sure analysis.
- It is to be used and adopted for routine use.
- It provides strong attachment of section to the slide, even for fat tissues.

Procedure

After obtaining biopsy specimen it is transferred to frozen section lab. Tissue is embedded on the metal chuck with the use of commercial preparation. For freezing, metal chuck is placed in stainless steel box containing aluminum racks, around which dry ice is packed. Cylindrical cavities are filled with 95% ethyl alcohol. Metal chuck containing specimen is inserted into one of the cavities. 15–20 seconds are required to freeze a block of tissue. After freezing, the tissue is placed in microtome and sections are cut at 6–8 μm for fixation. The slides with tissue attached are next immersed for few sec in solution composed of equal parts of Ether and Ethyl alcohol and stained with H and E staining. Stained sections are mounted and retained for permanent reference. Time required is 10 minutes. The exact report is recorded by the pathologist on 'Frozen section diagnosis form.'

Sialochemical Investigations

Saliva is a unique fluid and as a diagnostic fluid, it offers distinctive advantages over serum since it can be collected noninvasively by individual with modest training. Saliva may provide a cost-effective approach for the screening of oral lesions in a large population. Sialochemical investigations may be useful for diagnosis of hereditary, autoimmune, malignant and infectious diseases and endocrine disorders, as well as in the assessment of therapeutic levels of various drugs and monitoring of illicit drug use.

Advances in sialochemical diagnosis have been tremendously affected by current technological developments, such as the ability to measure and monitor a wide range of molecular components in saliva and compare them to serum components has made it feasible to study microbes, chemicals and immunologic markers. Large numbers of pediatricians, endocrinologists, immunologists, pharmacologists, clinical pathologists and dentists have found oral fluids as an easily available, noninvasive diagnostic medium for a wide range of diseases, clinical situations and field studies. Saliva lacks the drama of blood, the sincerity of sweat and emotional appeal of tears.

Examination of individual gland secretions can serve as a valuable adjunct in the differential diagnosis of local diseases and salivary gland dysfunctions. In case of autoimmune disease such as Sjögren's syndrome and graft v/s host disease, salivary flow rate measurement and analysis of specific components can serve as a screening test to determine whether labial gland or major salivary gland biopsy is indicated.

Saliva collected by expectoration or by special 'dip stick' techniques monitors' *Streptococcus mutans* and lactobacilli in tests currently being used to identify children at high-risk for dental caries and older adults susceptible to root caries. Quantization of *Candida albicans* from whole saliva can indicate infection. Host cell products derived from gingival sulcular fluid and admixing saliva have the potential in diagnosis of periodontal disease. The value of oral fluids in screening for HIV infection cannot be ruled out and is now being used in many field trials and epidemiological studies. Salivary monitoring can also be applied to diagnosing rubella, hepatitis A and B infection. Other recent salivary diagnosis includes tests for the presence of cysticocercosis and measuring specific IgA antibodies to gliadin as a marker for coelic disease. It also helps in evaluation of patients with diseases like cystic fibrosis, renal failure, Addison's disease, primary aldosteronism as a cause of hypertension and heavy metal intoxication. Research on viral isolation, immunoglobulin concentrations and taste dysfunction are also being developed.

Saliva reflects the issue fluid levels of natural substances a large variety of molecules have been introduced for therapeutic, dependency or recreational purpose. It represents the emotional status from high anxiety to low moods due to stress and depression. It shows the immunological status, responsiveness, neurological, nutritional status of the patient and metabolic influences of the patient. Sialochemical investigations are preferred by children and patients with limited coping abilities, such as the elderly. It is economical and patients can collect samples themselves saving technicians time. The saliva samples can be collected by either of the two mentioned methods:

1. *Gland specific saliva:* It is collected from the individual glands, parotid, submandibular and sublingual glands. Specimens of parotid and mixed submandibular-sublingual glands are collected with small cups held to the orifice by light suction. The minor salivary glands are distributed throughout the mouth except gingiva and anterior region of hard palate. Any secretion draining from mouth can be from minor salivary gland. Gland specific saliva is useful for detection of gland specific pathology, i.e. infection and obstruction.
2. *Whole saliva or mixed saliva:* It is a mixture of oral fluids and includes secretions from both major and minor salivary glands. In addition, to several constituents of nonsalivary origin such as gingival sulcular fluid, expectorated bronchial and nasal secretions, serum and blood derivatives from oral wounds, bacteria, and bacterial products, viruses and fungi, desquamated epithelial cells, other cellular components and food debris, it is also used for evaluation of systemic diseases.

   Stimulated saliva is collected by masticatory action or by gustatory stimulation. Stimulation affects the quantity of saliva; the concentrations of some constituents and the pH of the fluid. Unstimulated saliva is collected without exogenous gustatory, masticatory or mechanical stimulation. Its flow rate is affected by the degree of hydration, olfactory stimulation, exposure to light, body positioning, seasonal and diurnal factors.

   Whole saliva can be collected by either draining method in which saliva is allowed to drip off the lower lip or the spitting method where the subject expectorates saliva into test tubes. Serum constituents present in whole saliva is due to the GCF outflow. Depending upon degree of inflammation in gingiva, GCF is either serum transudate or more commonly an inflammatory exudate that contains serum constituents. Within the salivary glands, transfer mechanisms include intracellular and extracellular routes.

The sialochemical investigations are useful in the following:

- In determining the caries activity by various caries activity tests in children and older individual.

- In determination of oral candidiasis in denture wearers, immunocompromised patients, patients receiving various therapy and medications and in HIV infections.
- In periodontitis cases.
- In evaluation of various systemic diseases such as rheumatic arthritis, systemic sclerosis, graft v/s host disease, systemic lupus erythemateus (SLE), cystic fibrosis, hypertension, hyperlipidemia, alcoholic cirrhosis, diabetes mellitus, pancreatitis, adrenal-cortical disease, thyroiditis and acromegaly, parkinsonium, Bell's palsy and cerebral palsy.
- It can also be used as a diagnostic aid for digitalis toxicity, stomatitis with cancer therapy, gastric ulcer and ovulation time.
- It can also be used in monitoring certain drugs such as antipyrine, caffeine, carbamazepine, quinine, cisplastin, cyclosporine, metronidazole, paracetamol, diazepam, digoxin, ethosuximide, methadone, metoprolol, oxprenolol, primidone, procainamide, sulfanilamide, theophylline and tolbutamide.
- It is also helpful in identifying various drugs such as amphetamines, barbiturates, benzodiazepines, marijuana, nicotine, opioids and phencyclidine in drug abuse cases.
- It can also be administered in monitoring of cortisol and prednisone in Cushing's disease and Addison's disease, estrogen and progesterone in pregnancy and menstrual disturbances and insulin monitoring in diabetes mellitus.
- Saliva can be used in diagnosing viral infections such as hepatitis A, B and C, HIV infection (IgG levels), mumps, measles, and rubella, HSV-1 in Bell's palsy, cytomegalovirus, Epstein-Barr virus, salivary antidengue IgM and IgG in dengue.
- P^{53} is a tumor suppressor protein, whose absence in saliva can be used as screening for tumor. Increased levels of salivary defensin I is seen in oral squamous cell carcinoma. Tumor markers namely C-erb B-2, cancer Ag 15-3 may be present in saliva of females with breast cancer and CA 125 can be seen in epithelial ovarian cancer.
- Sialochemical findings may also detect *Helicobacter pylori* in peptic ulcer disease and chronic gastritis and pneumococcal C-polysaccharide in pneumococcal pneumonia.

Serology

Serology is the study of serum to diagnose infectious disease by observing the immune antibody (Ab) produced by the entry of the antigen (Ag) or pathogen into the body. It is the study of Ag-Ab or immunological reaction of body. When we are exposed to bacteria or viruses (antigens), the body's immune system produces specific antibodies against the organism. Antibody levels (antibody titer) help physicians to determine whether an infection occurred recently, or occurred years ago. Serological investigations help in diagnosis of certain microbial diseases such as:

- Early diagnosis of diseases like TB, viral hepatitis, rheumatic fever, acute glomerular nephritis, differential diagnosis of various enteric fevers, etc.
- It is of special importance for those organisms which are difficult to isolate and culture like syphilis, viral hepatitis.
- It is useful in measuring Ab levels to determine prevalence, spread and control of infectious disease.

The various types of serological tests include:

- *Precipitation reaction:* It is of the following types:
  - *Ring test:* For example C-reactive protein, streptococcal grouping.
  - *Flocculation test:* It is of 2 types: slide test (e.g. VDRL) and tube test.
  - Immunodiffusion test.
- *Agglutination test:* It is of the following types:
  - *Slide test:* For example *Salmonella* species blood grouping
  - *Tube test:* Typhoid (Widal test), brucellosis, typhus fever (Weil-Felix reaction)
  - *Antiglobulin (Coombs) test:* This is used for anti Rh Ab, incomplete Ab brucellosis
  - *Heterophile test:*
    - i. Weil-Felix test for *Proteus* strain, rickettsial species
    - ii. Paul-Bunnell test for infectious mononucleosis
    - iii. *Streptococcus* MG test for atypical pneumonia.
  - *Passive test:*
    - i. Latex agglutination test for hepatitis B, ASO, C-reactive protein, rheumatoid arthritis factor
    - ii. Hemagglutination for rheumatoid arthritis factor
    - iii. Coagglutination for *Streptococcus pyogenes* and *H. influenzae.*
  - *Widal test:* This test is performed for the diagnosis of typhoid and paratyphoid fever. The specific antibodies are usually detectable in the patients' blood, after 6 days of enteric fever, when the laboratory culture may not yield useful information. Serum sample of a typhi patient is tested for 'O' and 'H' antibodies by using antigenic suspensions, *Salmonella typhi* 'O' and *Salmonella typhi* 'H', respectively. In typhoid fever an increase in the agglutinations (titre above 240) is observed. For paratyphoid testing, the antigen suspensions used are *S. paratyphi* 'AH' and *S. paratyphi* 'BH'.
- **Complement fixation test**
- *Neutralization test:* It can be *in vivo* and *in vitro*. The *in vivo* tests are of the following types:
  - Toxigenicity test for *C. diphtheriae*
  - Shick test for diphtheria toxin.

  The in vitro tests are:
  - Antistreptolysin (ASO) titer for *Streptococcus pyogenes*
  - Virus neutralization test for typing viral isolate.
- *Immunofluorescence:* There are wide ranges of immunological tests available to assist in the diagnosis of diseases affecting oral cavity. These have now become an essential part of the diagnostic processes of the oral

medicine. Ag and Ab complexes are evaluated in dark field microscope. It is either direct for bacteria, virus, rabies or indirect. Many lesions of the oral mucosa are difficult to diagnose on clinical grounds and in some cases, the diagnosis may still be uncertain after conventional histopathological examination. It is important that such lesions be accurately diagnosed because they respond to different forms of treatment, may be associated with different systemic problems and may have differential prognosis.

Immunofluorescent technique has been used for 40 years to localize antigenically distinct molecules in tissue sections for microscopy. This is achieved by the use of specific antibody which when prepared appropriately, is used to detect substantial differences at the molecular level. The combination of antibody with its specific antigen does not lead to a visible change and therefore a readily identifiable label must be irreversibly found to the antibody so that its localization can be recognized. Immunofluorescence combines immunologic methods and histochemical methods to demonstrate the presence of an antigen or antibody in tissue, in serum or an organism.

The immunofluorescence assays are sensitive and reliable. Minute concentrations of antibodies and of soluble protein antigen can be detected. In concentrate of $10^{-4}/mL^3$, moreover insoluble antigens in tissue can be tested for directly by using immunofluorescence.

Immunofluorescence can be used for identification of T-and B-cells in blood, detection of autoantibodies is serum, immunoglobulin and complement components in tissues, specific tissue fixed Ab, identification of microorganisms, tumor specific antigen on neoplastic tissue, transplantation Ag in various organs, chromosome, localization of hormones and enzyme and quantization of sperm protein and Ab's.

- **Radioimmuno assay**
- *Enzyme-linked immunosorbent assay (ELISA):* It is used for HIV, tuberculosis, rotavirus, hepatitis B and *E.coli*. It is the more popular and widely done test for diagnosis of HIV. It is a test with 99% specificity and sensitivity, especially on repeated testing. ELISA is a test that uses antibodies and color change to identify a substance. It is cheaper than polymerase chain reaction (PCR) and culture and hence is the mainstay of HIV diagnosis in developing countries. In developed countries, however, western blot test is necessary if ELISA is positive, to confirm a person as HIV-positive. ELISA is negative in the window period, that is, 6–12 weeks following HIV exposure and in newborn. One will have to wait for 18 months to diagnose HIV infection in newborn if one uses only ELISA. ELISA can also be used in toxicology as a rapid presumptive screen for certain classes of drugs. Dr Dennis E Bidwell and Alister Voller created the ELISA test to detect various kinds of diseases, such as malaria, Chagas disease, and Johne's disease. ELISA tests also are used as *in vitro* diagnostics in medical laboratories. The other uses of ELISA include detection of *Mycobacterium* antibodies in tuberculosis, rotavirus in feces, hepatitis B markers in serum and enterotoxin of *E. coli* in feces.

It is of the following types:

- Indirect ELISA
- Sandwich or direct ELISA
- Competitive ELISA
- Multiple and portable ELISA.

Cytogenetics and Chromosome Analysis

Normal human somatic cells contain 46 chromosomes. They can be demonstrated only in actively dividing cells by mitosis. In metaphase the chromosomes are distinct and stainable. They can be easily counted and classified. Usually, cells from bone marrow, testis, and tumors are preferred because rapid division is occurring. Small lymphocytes of blood can be stimulated to divide by phytohemagglutinin and preparations rich in metaphase cells can be obtained by culturing lymphocytes cells with colchicine or vinblastine sulfate.

Chromosome analysis is only a gross tool to investigate genetic diseases. Many genetic differences among individuals are observable by chemical analysis of body tissues. Genetic abnormalities are reflected in chromosome abnormality, such as:

Aneuploidy which is defined as the abnormal number of chromosomes in all the cells of an individual. It occurs due to error in meiosis. It is seen in Klinefelter's syndrome in male having 47 XXY or 48 XXXY karyotype, in Turner's syndrome: 45 XO karyotype and Down syndrome 47 XY in male (Mongolism).

Structural variations can be due to translocations, deletions, inversions and rings. Abnormalities in the number and size of X chromosome can also made by counting Barr bodies (1 μ in size). It is used in diagnosing cases with Turner's disease. Barr body in one of two X chromosome of female is seen when at least 2 X chromosomes are there.

Large number of chromosomal abnormalities has been seen to be associated with oral anomalies like oral clefts, palatal vaulting, mandibular hypoplasia or prognathism or dental agenesis. Down's syndrome or Trisomy 21 is shown to be associated with chronic myelogenous leukemia. Chromosomal abnormality has also been associated with lymphomas, malignancies and as a result of herpes simplex or other viral infections.

Maxillofacial Imaging

The role of imaging in oral medicine varies greatly with the type of problem being evaluated. Certain problems, such as pain in the orofacial region, frequently require imaging to determine the origin of the pain. For other conditions, however, such as soft-tissue lesions of the oral mucosa, imaging offers no new diagnostic information. The variety of imaging techniques available to the clinician has grown in number and in degree of sophistication over the years. While this means that there is an imaging procedure that will provide the information desired by the clinician, it also means that choosing the best technique is not necessarily an easy process.

The decision to order diagnostic imaging as part of the evaluation of an orofacial complaint should be based on the history obtained from the patient, clinical examination, and then determine both the type of additional information required (if any) and the best technique for obtaining this information. There are many reasons for requesting imaging information, including the determination of the nature of a condition, the confirmation of a clinical diagnosis, the evaluation of the extent of a lesion, and the monitoring of the progression or regression of a lesion over time. Each of these may require a different imaging strategy.

Whether or not there are certain guidelines for selecting the imaging technique, it is incumbent upon the clinician to wisely use diagnostic imaging. This means the clinician should specifically determine what information is needed, deciding whether imaging is the best way to obtain this information, and (if so) selecting the most appropriate technique, after considering the information needed, the radiation dose and cost, the availability of the technique, and the skills needed to interpret the study.

Various imaging modalities are available in the dental clinics and offices and in hospitals and radiology clinics. They can be broadly grouped as under:

- Intraoral imaging
- Extraoral imaging.

Intraoral Imaging

There are a number of imaging modalities that are readily available to the clinician for evaluating patients' conditions. Virtually every dental office has the equipment to perform intraoral radiography. Intraoral radiographic examinations are the backbone of imaging for the general dentist. The advantage of intraoral radiography is the fine detail provided in its visualization of the teeth and supporting bone. Intraoral radiographs can be divided into three categories: periapical, bitewing and occlusal radiographs. When intraoral digital image receptors are used, the radiographic principles are the same as those for radiographic films. The various intraoral projections are discussed below:

- *Periapical radiographs:* They should show all of a tooth, including the surrounding bone. Two projection techniques are commonly used for periapical radiography, the paralleling technique and the bisecting angle technique. Most clinicians prefer the paralleling technique as it provides a less distorted view of the dentition.

  The paralleling technique, also called the right-angle or long-cone technique is based on the principle that the X-ray film is supported parallel to the long axis of the teeth and the central ray of the X-ray beam is directed at right angles to the teeth and film. It was given by F G Fitzgerald in 1947.

  The bisecting angle technique is based on the Cieszynski's rule of isometry, which states that 2 triangles are equal when they share one complete side and have 2 equal angles.

The periapical radiography is indicated for the following:
- Detection of apical infection/inflammation
- Evaluation of periodontal condition
- Evaluation of unerupted teeth
- Assessment of trauma to teeth and alveolar bone
- Assessment of root canal morphology during endodontic treatment and root morphology before extractions
- Evaluation of lesions within alveolar bone and evaluation of implants
- Preoperative and postoperative assessment of apical surgery

  Periapical films are available as:
  No. 0 for children (22 × 35 mm)
  No. 1 for anterior adult projections (24 × 40 mm)
  No. 2 for posterior adult projections (31 × 41 mm)

- *Bitewing radiographs:* These show only the crowns of the teeth and the adjacent alveolar crests. This technique was perfected by Howard Raper in 1924-25. These films have a paper tab projecting from the middle of the film on which the patient bites to support the film. They help in the
  - Detection of interproximal caries and secondary caries especially at the pulpal and cervical floor
  - Study the proximity of carious lesions to pulp
  - Detection of early periodontal disease
  - Detection of calculus on proximal surface
  - Conduction of large scale radiographic surveys for prevalence of dental caries and periodontal disease
  - To check the gingival fit of Class II restorations.

  Bitewing films are available as:
  Size 0 for child (posterior) (22 × 35 mm)
  Size 1 for child (anterior) (24 × 40 mm)
  Size 2 for adult (posterior) (31 × 41 mm)
  Size 3 for adult (anterior) (27 × 54 mm)

- *Occlusal radiographs:* These radiographs show an area of teeth and bone larger than periapical radiographs. The film as available as size 2 (57 × 76 mm). Occlusal radiography is of 2 types namely, cross-sectional and topographic. These are typically indicated in the following cases:
  - To localize roots, supernumerary, unerupted and impacted teeth
  - To localize foreign bodies in the jaws and stones in the ducts of sublingual and submandibular glands
  - To study changes in buccal and lingual cortical plates, buccolingual extent of pathoses and displacement, location, nature and extent of fracture lines
  - To study large lesions, that cannot be seen completely on periapical radiographs
  - To determine the medial and lateral extent of cysts, tumors, osteomyelitis, etc. and to detect any diseases in the palate and floor of the mouth

- To aid in the examination of patients with trismus, patients who are unable to open their mouth wide enough for periapical radiographs or for other reasons cannot accept periapical radiography.

Extraoral Imaging

The X-ray source and image receptor are placed outside the patient's mouth in extraoral radiographic examinations. Extraoral films commonly used in dentistry are of sizes 5" × 7", 8" × 10", as well as panoramic, 5" × 12" and 6" × 12". These include the following projections:

- *Panoramic radiography:* Panoramic radiography demonstrates a wide view of the maxilla and mandible as well as surrounding structures, including the neck, temporomandibular joint (TMJ), zygomatic arches, maxillary sinuses and nasal cavity, and orbits although it does so with less sharpness and detail than are seen in intraoral views. It is a curvilinear variant of tomography which is based on the principle of reciprocal movement of the film and source around the central plane called as image layer. This is called focal trough which is 3-D curved zone located within the object whose image is seen clearly on the radiograph. The X-ray source rotates around 3 centers of rotation during scanning.

  Comparison of right and left sides is easier with a panoramic projection, and this view provides an excellent initial view of the osseous structures of the TMJ and of the integrity of the sinus floor. Additional views targeting these tissues can be obtained later if needed. Some panoramic X-ray machines also have the capability of providing a variety of skull projections, including lateral, oblique lateral, posteroanterior, anteroposterior, and submentovertex views. Typically, these are done with a cephalometric attachment to the machine. Although these views are relatively easy to take and can provide valuable information in certain circumstances, they demonstrate complex anatomy and should be interpreted by an oral and maxillofacial radiologist. It is indicated for the following:
  - To evaluate trauma cases from fracture and dislocation
  - To study and locate impacted, supernumerary and unerupted teeth
  - To study developmental anomalies affecting the teeth, jaws and growth of the jaws
  - To study the alignment of teeth for orthodontic purposes
  - To study the temporomandibular joint (TMJ) and the maxillary sinus
  - To study parotid sialographs
  - To assess the implant site and condition of alveolar ridges
  - To study large tumors and cysts that cannot be seen on periapical films.
- *Lateral oblique view:* It can be taken by regular intraoral X-ray machine. It is indicated for the examination of the following:
  - Gross examination of maxilla or mandible
  - Examination of patients with trismus and teeth and jaws of children who cannot tolerate intraoral films
  - To detect and locate impacted, supernumerary and unerupted teeth

  - To detect and locate cysts, tumors and other pathologies
  - To detect fracture lines.
- *True lateral view:* Unlike lateral view there is complete superimposition of right and left sides of the jaws in this view. It is indicated for the following:
  - To study fractures of nasal bone and maxilla
  - To study the posterior wall of maxillary sinus
  - To study cysts, tumors and malignancies in the maxillary antrum
  - To localize any foreign bodies
  - To study hair on end appearance in thalassemia
  - To study the multiple punched out radiolucencies in multiple myeloma, metastatic malignancies and eosinophilic granuloma and the cotton wool appearance of Paget's disease.
- *PA Caldwell's view:* It is indicated for the gross examination of maxilla and mandible, to study large lesions of the jaws, study fracture lines of mandible alongwith displacement and to study fracture of skull bones.
- *PA Water's view:* This view is indicated for the following:
  - To study maxillary sinus
  - To study fractures involving middle third of the facial skeleton, zygomatic arches and orbits
  - To study frontal and ethmoidal sinuses
  - To study coronoid process
  - To study deviated nasal septum.
- *PA rotated view:* This is used to study calculus in parotid duct and displacement of condyles.
- *Reverse Towne's view:* It is employed to study the condylar fracture and displacement and study the continuity of zygomatic arches.

Temporomandibular Joint Radiography

Temporomandibular joint (TMJ) imaging may be necessary to supplement information obtained from the clinical examination, particularly when an osseous abnormality or infection is suspected, failure of conservative treatment or worsening of the symptoms is observed. It should also be considered in patients with a history of trauma, alteration in the range of movements, marked dysfunction, sensory or motor abnormalities or significant changes in occlusion of the patient. The purpose of this imaging is to evaluate the integrity and relationships of the hard and soft tissues, confirm the extent or stage of progression of the disease and evaluate the treatment effects. The practitioner must correlate the radiographic findings with patient's history and clinical observation to formulate a final diagnosis and plan the treatment.

The type of imaging technique selected depends on the specific clinical problem, whether imaging of hard or soft tissues is desired, the amount of diagnostic information available form a particular imaging technique, cost and radiation dose. The TMJ imaging is divided as hard tissue and soft tissue imaging.

Hard Tissue Imaging

- **Panoramic projection:** It serves as a screening technique to identify odontogenic diseases and other conditions that may be a source of TMJ symptoms. Gross changes in the condyles may be identified, like large osteophytes, asymmetries, fractures or extensive erosions.
- **Transcranial projection (Lindblom's view):** It is used to study the following:
  - Position of the condyle in glenoid fossa
  - Study joint space for either partial or complete obliteration
  - Study anteroposterior mobility (hypermobility, i.e. dislocation and subluxation)
  - Study osseous changes such as flattening in arthritis.
- **Transpharyngeal projection/Parma projection (McQuein's projection):** It is indicated to study the following:
  - Head and neck of condyle
  - Flattening of condyle in rheumatoid arthritis and osteophytes in osteoarthritis
  - Elongated styloid process
  - Fractures involving neck of condyle
  - Developmental abnormalities affecting the condyle
  - Parotid gland sialography.
- **Transorbital projection (Zimmer's projection):** This is an antero-posterior view, indicated to study:
  - Mediolateral displacement of condyle
  - Superior surface of condyle for osteophytes
  - Relationship of condyle to articular eminence in mediolateral plane.
- **Submento vertex view:** This projection provides a view of the skull base and condyles superimposed on the condyle necks and mandibular rami. It is used as an adjunct to views depicting the TMJs in the lateral plane. This view is used to study the fractures of zygomatic arch, posterior wall of maxillary sinus, fractures involving the base of skull and to study the sphenoidal air sinus.
- **Conventional tomography:** Plain (or conventional) tomography is a radiographic technique that has been available for many years, generally in institutions such as dental schools or hospitals, due to the size and expense of the equipment. However, tomographic capability has been added to some sophisticated computer-controlled panoramic X-ray machines, making tomography potentially more readily available in dental offices and clinics. It has been used for detailed evaluation of the osseous structures of the TMJ in the past. It is desirable to supplement this examination with frontal tomographs, particularly when morphologic abnormalities or erosive changes of the condylar head are suspected.
- **Computed tomography:** Computed tomography (CT) permits the imaging of thin slices of tissue in a wide variety of planes. Most CT is done in the axial plane, and many CT scans also provide coronal views; sagittal slices are

less commonly used. During CT scanning, the X-ray source and detectors move around the desired region of the body while the patient lies on a table. It is indicated when more information is needed about the 3-dimensional shape and internal structure of the osseous components of the joint or if information regarding the surrounding soft tissues is required.

CT is typically used in dentistry to evaluate:

- The extent of lesions suspected or detected with other radiographic techniques
- The degree of maxillofacial involvement in cases of trauma
- The integrity and condition of the paranasal sinuses
- The quality and quantity of bone in proposed dental implant sites, particularly when there are multiple sites or when there has been bone grafting.

Computed tomography (CT) is rarely indicated for evaluation of the TMJ since the osseous structures can be visualized adequately with less expensive techniques such as conventional tomography or panoramic radiography, and disk displacement and other joint soft-tissue information can be better obtained with magnetic resonance imaging. CT may be of value in complex TMJ situations, such as in cases of suspected ankylosis or severe joint destruction or when there is a history of polytetrafluoroethylene or silicon-sheeting TMJ implants which may cause complications such as erosions into the middle cranial fossa and heterotropic bone growth.

Soft Tissue Imaging

The soft tissues can be imaged with magnetic resonance imaging (MRI) or arthrography. These should only be used when information about the condition of the soft tissue components is required for treatment planning. Arthrography is indicated when information about disk position, morphology, function and integrity of diskal attachments is required for planning the treatment. Arthrography is invasive and technically difficult and has been replaced by MRI in most institutions. MRI can indicate a pathologic condition of the soft tissue through altered tissue signal, allowing evaluation of the disk and surrounding muscles, and can image joint effusion. It is more expensive and contraindicated in pregnant women, patients with pacemakers, intracranial vascular clips or metal particles in vital structures.

Ultrasonography

Ultrasonography (USG) uses the reflection of sound waves to provide information about tissues and their interfaces with other tissues. This is a noninvasive and relatively inexpensive technique for imaging superficial tissues in "real time." The operator applies a probe over the area of interest and receives information immediately on the computer monitor. In regard to the head and neck region, there has been a great deal of recent interest in the imaging of salivary glands. Several researchers have studied the ultrasonographic features of a variety of tumors and other conditions in the parotid gland, in an attempt to make a diagnosis before biopsy as the surgical management of these tumors may vary. Others have looked at the heterogeneity of sonic echo production within the parenchyma of parotid glands affected by a variety of inflammatory or autoimmune conditions. Efforts are being made to categorize lymph nodes in the neck as metastatic, reactive, or normal in patients with head and neck neoplasms. Unfortunately, USG does not appear to be useful for determining internal derangement of the TMJ at this time although work is continuing in this area.

Nuclear Medicine

In radionuclide imaging (nuclear medicine, scintigraphy), a substance labeled with a radioactive isotope is injected intravenously. Depending on the specific material used, the substance will be taken up preferentially by the thyroid (technetium [Tc] 99m-labeled iodine), salivary glands (Tc 99m pertechnetate), or bone (Tc 99m methylene diphosphonate [MDP]). Gallium 67 citrate is also sometimes used to assess infections and inflammation in bone. At various times after radionuclide injection, a gamma camera is used to count the radioactivity in the various organs and tissues of the body and to display the results visually. High concentrations of the isotope show up as "hot spots" and generally indicate high metabolic activity.

Nuclear-medicine scans are used to assess conditions that may be widespread, such as metastasis to bone or other tissues or such as fibrous dysplasia in an active phase. Unfortunately, areas of dental periapical and periodontal inflammation also take up the tracer, presenting as hot spots in the jaws, and must be differentiated from other pathologic conditions. A variation of bone scintigraphy that can be used to localize and quantify bone activity is single-photon emission computed tomography (SPECT). Volumetric measurements may also be obtained to quantify the distribution of radioactivity in the tissue, allowing better assessment of tissue function. A recent study demonstrated the use of SPECT in the evaluation of osseointegration in dental implants. However, in another study, both the sensitivity and specificity of SPECT were low for the detection of painful sites in patients with idiopathic jaw pain.

Imaging for Salivary Gland Diseases

Plain films are used to study stones in the salivary glands. The parotid glands can be studied with OPG, lateral oblique view and AP view. The stones of the submandibular glands can be studied with true occlusal view of the mandible, OPG or a lateral oblique view.

Sialography

It is one of the oldest modality to study the salivary ductal system. It was described by Capry in 1902. In this technique, a radiopaque dye is injected into the ducts of the glands and a radiographic image is obtained. It is indicated in the following cases:

- To study radiolucent sialoliths
- To study the extent of destruction of the duct due to the stone or a foreign body
- To study recurrent inflammations of the gland
- To study and diagnose fistulas and diverticuli
- To outline the plane of facial nerve prior to biopsies
- To demonstrate a tumor, its size, location and extent
- Therapeutic dilatation of strictures by forceful injection of the dye.

It is contraindicated in patients who are allergic to the contrast media being used, patients with acute salivary gland infections and those who are scheduled to undergo thyroid function test.

Five Steps

1. Clinical examination
2. Preliminary radiographic examination
3. Cannulation of the duct
4. Injection of contrast media
5. *Phases of sialography:* Ductal phase, acinar phase and evacuation phase.

Sialographic appearances in various diseases are as under:

- *Sialoliths:* Filling defect with segmental strictures and retention of the contrast media on the sialogram
- *Sialodochitis:* Segmental stricture of the ducts gives rise to a sausage string appearance
- *Sjögren's syndrome:* Cherry blossom or branchless fruit laden tree appearance
- *Sialoadenitis:* Apple tree like appearance
- *Benign tumors:* Ball in hand appearance
- Ductal irregularity with abnormal contrast puddling on a sialogram is suggestive of a malignant tumor of the salivary gland.

Radionuclide canning/scintigraphy may be done using Tc 99m pertechnetate. This technique is mainly indicated when sialography cannot be performed in ductal obstructions/sialoliths, to study salivary gland aplasia, tumors of salivary gland and study and diagnose Sjögren's syndrome. MRI scans also may be used to study tumors of the gland and Sjögren's syndrome. USG can be used to study sialoliths, cyst and tumors within the salivary gland.

7

Therapeutics

Commonly Used Drugs in Dentistry

Drug	*Aspirin*
Comments	*Mild analgesic*: Not usually termed as NSAID. Management of pain with significant inflammatory component, musculoskeletal pain, headache, antipyretic, and in prophylaxis of cardiovascular disease (CVD) and myocardial infarction (MI) due to its antiplatelet actions Hepatotoxic in overdose or prolonged use. Causes aspirin burn, gastric ulcers, is uricosuric and can precipitate gout. It should not be prescribed to asthmatics, children <12 years of age, patients with uncontrolled hypertension and patients with disorders of hemostasis.
Dose	Analgesia and antipyretic 300–900 mg QID/TID Antiplatelet action 75–300 mg per day

Drug	*Aceclofenac*
Comments	*Analgesic for moderate pain*: NSAID Pain and inflammation associated with musculoskeletal disorders such as rheumatoid arthritis, osteoarthritis and ankylosing spondylitis. Post-operative pain Ibuprofen and aspirin should be avoided in these patients due to increase in unwanted effects, especially gastrointestinal (GI) ulceration, renal and liver damage.
Dose	100 mg tablet OD

Drug	*Diclofenac*
Comments	*Analgesic for moderate pain*: NSAID Pain and inflammation associated with musculoskeletal disorders such as rheumatoid arthritis, osteoarthritis and ankylosing spondylitis. Post-operative pain Contraindicated in peptic ulcer, aspirin sensitivity and pregnancy. To be given with caution in elderly, renal, liver or cardiac disease
Dose	25–75 mg up to twice daily

Drug	*Ibuprofen*
Comments	Management of pain with significant inflammatory component, musculoskeletal pain, dysmenorrheal and antipyretic Contraindicated in peptic ulcer, aspirin sensitivity and asthmatics or patients with history of angioedema and urticaria or patients with hemorrhagic disorders.
Dose	Adults 1.2–1.8 g daily in divided doses Children 20–40 mg/kg

Drug	*Paracetamol*
Comments	Mild-to-moderate pain and as antipyretic. Hepatotoxicity in overdose, avoid in renal failure patients and those with alcohol abuse.
Dose	Adults 0.5–1 g QID/TID Children 3 months–1 year, 60–120 mg every 4–6 hours 1–5 years, 120–150 mg every 4–6 hours 6–12 years, 250–500 mg every 4–6 hours

Drug	*Acyclovir*
Comments	Antiviral, used in treatment of herpes simplex and varicella zoster infections. May reduce effect of anticonvulsant drugs, increase toxicity of pethidine. Probenecid increases its plasma concentration.
Dose	Adults 200–400 mg 5 times a day (or topical application), children under 2 years should be given half the adult dose

Drug	*Epinephrine*
Comments	Used in dental anesthesia to increase efficacy and duration and aid in hemostasis Excessive dosage may produce tachycardia and tremors. Systolic BP may rise and diastolic may fall. May cause cardiac arrhythmias.
Dose	It is contained in the LA solutions in concentrations of 1:80,000, 1:100,000, and 1:200,000. Maximum recommended dose over a single visit is 200 g.

Drug	*Amoxicillin*
Comments	Broad-spectrum beta-lactam antibacterial To treat bacterial infection such as dental abscess and as prophylactic in prevention of infective endocarditis. Reduces efficacy of oral contraceptives, reduces excretion of methotrexate. Its activity is decreased by tetracyclines and probenecid increases its half-life. It may induce glossitis and tongue discoloration and candidiasis

Dose	*For dental infections*: 250-500 mg TID for outpatient treatment, 500–1,000 mg IV QID for severe infections and 50% of adult dose in children under 10 years *For prophylaxis*: 2 g every one hour preoperatively when treated under LA Children under 5 years 25% of adult dose and in 5–10 years 50% of adult dose.

Drug	*Ampicillin*
Comments	Broad-spectrum beta-lactam antibacterial To treat bacterial infection such as dental abscess Reduces efficacy of oral contraceptives, reduces excretion of methotrexate. Its activity is decreased by tetracyclines and probenecid increases its half-life. It may induce glossitis and tongue discoloration and candidiasis
Dose	250–1,000 mg QID and 50% of adult dose in children under 10 years

Drug	*Amphotericin*
Comments	Antifungal used to treat candidal infections. Contraindicated in GI disturbances, renal damage. Its action is decreased during combined therapy with fluconazole, ketoconazole and miconazole.
Dose	Available as 100 mg tablets, 10 mg lozenges, 100 mg/ml oral suspension

Drug	*Penicillin G/Penicillin V*
Comments	Most oral bacterial infections such as abscess
Dose	Adult, 500 mg QID Child, under 6 years 25% of adult dose and 50% of adult dose in 6–12 years

Drug	*Augmentin (co-amoxiclav)*
Comments	Mixture of amoxicillin and potassium clavulanate Inhibits some penicillinases and therefore active against *Staphylococcus aureus* Inhibits some lactamases and is therefore active against some gram-negative and penicillin resistant bacteria Contraindicated in penicillin hypersensitivity and in hepatic patients
Dose	125/250 mg TID

Drug	Benzyl penicillin
Comments	Broad-spectrum beta-lactam antibacterial To treat bacterial infection such as dental abscess Most effective penicillin where organism sensitive Contraindicated in penicillin hypersensitivity
Route	Oral or IM
Dose	Adult, 600 mg–1.2 g QID Child, 1–12 years 100–300 mg/kg daily in 4–6 doses

Drug	*Tetracyclines*
Comments	Broad-spectrum antibacterial, but rarely indicated for dental infections except in periodontal disease. Cause discoloration of developing teeth and have absorption impaired by iron, antacids, milk, etc. Use may predispose to cardiosis and to nausea and gastrointestinal disturbance Contraindicated in pregnancy and children at least up to 8 years Frequent mild gastrointestinal effects
Dose	250–500 mg QID daily to treat dental infections. When used in the management of periodontal disease the duration of therapy is 2 weeks.

Drug	*Doxycycline*
Comments	Broad-spectrum tetracycline used occasionally in the treatment of sinusitis. Cause discoloration of developing teeth and have absorption impaired by iron, antacids, milk, etc. Use may predispose to cardiosis and to nausea and gastrointestinal disturbance, Stevens-Johnson syndrome. Contraindicated in pregnancy and children at least up to 8 years Frequent mild gastrointestinal effects
Dose	200 mg on the first day, then 100 mg once daily

Drug	*Metronidazole*
Comments	Anerobic bacterial infections such as dental abscess, acute pericoronitis and acute ulcerative gingivitis. High doses contraindicated in pregnancy and during breastfeeding, avoid in hypersensitive patients and avoid alcohol (disulfiram like reaction). It may increase warfarin effect.
Dose	400 mg orally TID for 7 days or 500 mg BD IV daily

Drug	*Vancomycin*
Comments	Prophylaxis of endocarditis in those having a GA and who cannot receive amoxicillin. Contraindicated in pregnancy and during breastfeeding, renal disease, history of deafness. It may cause nausea, rashes, tinnitus, deafness Rapid injection may cause 'red man' syndrome.
Dose	1 g IV by slow injection over 1 hour

Drug	*Cephalosporins*
Comments	Broad-spectrum, beta-lactam antibiotics, with few absolute indications for use in dentistry, although they may be effective against *Staphylococcus aureus*. Cefuroxime is occasionally used for surgical prophylaxis in oral and maxillofacial surgery. Hypersensitivity is the main side effect, disulfiram like reaction may occur with alcohol. Cefuroxime is less affected by penicillinases than other cephalosporins and is currently the preferred drug of the many available. Cefazolin increases anticoagulant effect of warfarin effect of cephalosporins is reduced in combined therapy with tetracyclines or erythromycin.
Dose	250 mg QID and for children a daily dose of 25 mg/kg (in divided doses)

Drug	*Cephadroxil*
Comments	Beta-lactam antibiotics, used to treat gram-positive and gram-negative bacterial infections. Candidiasis and glossitis may occur after prolonged use. May cause thrombocytopenia, agranulocytosis and anemia.
Dose	250 mg QID and for children a daily dose of 25 mg/kg (in divided doses)

Drug	*Cephalexin*
Comments	Beta-lactam antibiotics, occasionally used as an alternative to penicillin to treat dental infections in patients allergic to latter. Hypersensitivity is the main side effect. As with penicillin probenecid decreases the excretion of the cephalosporins.
Dose	250 mg QID and for children a daily dose of 25 mg/kg (in divided doses)

Drug	*Clindamycin*
Comments	Antibacterial drug, first choice for prophylaxis of endocarditis in those allergic to penicillin, occasionally used for dental infections in cases where the disease has progressed to bone, in those allergic to penicillin Hypersensitivity is the main side effect, contraindicated in diarrhea patients. Renal failure may occur, if used in combination with gentamicin.
Dose	150–300 mg QID and for children a daily dose of 3–6 mg/kg (in 4 divided doses)

Drug	*Benzocaine*
Comments	Intraoral topical anesthesia Avoid excess use in mouth as loss of tongue and pharynx sensation can reduce protection of airway. Contraindicated in patients with allergy to ester group. It can produce methemoglobinemia at high dose or as an idiosyncratic reaction.
Dose	Topical preparations in concentrations from 6–20%. Dosage recommendations as provided by the manufacturer.

Drug	*Bupivacaine*
Comments	Local anesthesia, especially long-lasting anesthesia after regional block injection. Contraindicated in patients allergic to amide local anesthetic. It is more cardiotoxic than lidocaine. Reduce dose in hepatic disease.
Dose	Recommended maximum dose is 1.3 mg/kg with an absolute ceiling of 90 mg

Drug	*Diazepam*
Comments	Used in dental sedation and preoperative anxiolysis and also indicated in the emergency treatment of epilepsy in the dental surgery. Contraindicated in severe respiratory and liver disease, porphyria. May produce xerostomia, respiratory depression, hypotension or visual disturbances. Avoid with CNS depressant drugs.
Dose	To treat anxiolysis 2 mg–10 mg TID As premedication for dental treatment 5-10 mg, 1–2 hours prior to the surgery

Drug	*Fluconazole*
Comments	Antifungal agent, used to treat oral fungal infections. Contraindicated in pregnancy and during breastfeeding, previous hypersensitivity, GI problems.
Dose	50–100 mg daily for 7–14 days

Drug	*Itraconazole*
Comments	Antifungal agent, used to treat oral fungal infections. Contraindicated in renal and hepatic disease, previous hypersensitivity, GI problems. Discontinue, if peripheral neuropathy occurs.
Dose	100 mg daily for 15 days

Drug	*Ketoconazole*
Comments	Antifungal agent, used to treat systemic fungal infections and severe resistant mucocutaneous candidiasis . It is more readily absorbed than miconazole and lead to nephrotoxicity. It may cause hypersensitivity reactions and GI disturbances.
Dose	200 mg daily for 14 days. In children 3 mg/kg daily.

Drug	*Lignocaine*
Comments	Local anesthesia (topical and by injection). Lignocaine with epinephrine is the gold standard LA for dental anesthesia. Contraindicated in patients allergic to amide local anesthetic, acute porphyria.
Dose	2.0 mL or 2.2 mL cartridges for injection of a 2 % solution. Recommended maximum dose is 4.4 mg/kg with an absolute ceiling of 300 mg

Drug	*Nystatin*
Comments	Treatment of candidal infections. Contraindicated in hypersensitivity.
Dose	Pastille containing 100,000 units, suspension containing 100,000 units/mL or ointment containing 100,000 units/g

Drug	*Ropivacaine*
Comments	Local anesthesia Contraindicated in patients allergic to amide local anesthetic, less cardiotoxic than bupivacine, may cause CNS toxicity at high dose.
Dose	No more than 30 ml of the 0.75% solution in a 70 kg adult (adjust for weight in children) when used as field block.

Drug	*Saliva substitute*
Comments	Contains carboxymethylcellulose, carmellose sodium, xylitol or sorbitol and salts may also be used. Indicated in symptomatic treatment of xerostomia.
Dose	Used as required on oral mucosa. Available as sprays, gels and lozenges.

Some Topical Corticosteroids (More Preparations that are Potent)

Drug	*Hydrocortisone hemisuccinate pellets*
Dose 6 hourly	2.5 mg
Comments	Dissolve in mouth close to lesions Use at early stage

Drug	*Triamcinolone acetonide in carmellose gelatin paste*
Dose 6 hourly	Apply thin layer
Comments	Adheres best to dry mucosa Affords mechanical protection Of little value on tongue or palate

Drug	*Betamethasone phosphate tablets*
Dose 6 hourly	0.5 mg as a mouthwash
Comments	More potent than preparations above but many produce adrenal suppression

Some Intralesional Corticosteroids

Drug	*Prednisolone sodium phosphate*
Dose	Up to 24 mg
Comments	Short acting

Drug	*Methylprednisolone acetate*
Dose	4–80 mg every 1–5 weeks
Comments	Also available with lignocaine

Drug	*Triamcinolone acetonide*
Dose	2–3 mg every 1–2 weeks
Comments	—

Drug	*Triamcinolone hexacetonide*
Dose	Up to 5 mg every 3–4 weeks
Comments	—

Some Intra-articular Corticosteroids

Drug	*Dexamethasone sodium phosphate*
Dose	0.4–5 mg at intervals of 3–21 days
Comments	More expensive than hydrocortisone acetate

Drug	*Hydrocortisone acetate*
Dose	5–50 mg
Comments	Usual preparation used

Antifibrinolytic Agents

Drug	E-amine caproic acid
Comments	Useful in some bleeding tendencies May cause nausea, diarrhea, dizziness, myalgia contraindicated in pregnancy, history of thromboembolism, renal disease
Adult dose	3 g 4–6 times daily

Drug	Tranexamic acid
Comments	As above but tranexamic acid is usually the preferred drug
Adult dose	1–1.5 gm BD/TID Slow injection of 1 g TID

Treatment of Common Oral Diseases

Actinomycosis

- *Systemic therapy:* Antibiotics
  Preferred: Penicillin G 18–24 million units IV/d × 2–6 weeks, then amoxicillin 500–750 mg TID/QID × 6–12 months; oral therapy alone may be adequate.
  Alternatives:
  Doxycycline 100 mg twice daily IV × 2–6 weeks, then 100 mg twice daily × 6–12 months.
  Erythromycin 500 mg four times a day × 6–12 months.
  Clindamycin 600 mg IV QID × 2–6 weeks, then 300 mg QID × 6–12 months.
  Other agents (limited data): Clarithromycin, azithromycin, imipenem, cefotaxime and ceftriaxone.
- Wide excision of infected tissue

Acute Herpetic Gingivostomatitis

- Systemic therapy
  Valacyclovir 500 mg BD × 10 days
  Acyclovir 400 mg 1 tablet 5 times daily × 10 days
- Fluids
- Analgesia

Acute Necrotizing Ulcerative Gingivitis

Topical therapy is all that most patients will require, with systemic antibiotics being required only for patients with systemic signs of infection.

- Antimicrobial treatment recommendations
  Amoxicillin 500 mg TID for 10 days plus metronidazole 250 mg TID for 10 days or
  Amoxicillin-clavulanate 500 mg/125 mg TID or 875 mg/125 mg BID for 10 days or

Clindamycin 150–300 mg TID for 10 days or
Doxycycline 100 mg BID for 10 days

- *Adjunctive therapy:* Saline rinses can help to speed resolution; oral rinses with a hydrogen peroxide 3% solution may be of benefit.
  Chlorhexidine 0.12% oral rinse 15 mL BID
  For human immunodeficiency virus (HIV) positive patients, consider nystatin rinse 5 mL QID or fluconazole 200 mg daily for 7–14 days.
  Patients with ANUG should be given topical anesthetic and NSAIDs, because pain control is very important in allowing the patient to perform good oral hygiene.

Angioedema

The goals of emergency treatment of angioedema are to prevent spontaneous eruption, to maintain a patent airway, if eruption does occur, and to stop progression of disease. Laryngeal edema may occur rapidly. In these cases, a definitive airway, such as an endotracheal tube or nasopharyngeal airway, should be established. If the airway cannot be effectively secured with an endotracheal tube, a surgical airway is indicated, usually in the form of an emergency cricothyrotomy. Life-threatening airway obstruction (if swelling occurs in the throat) and anaphylactic reactions are possible complications.

Treatment of angioedema includes histamine blockers (H1 and H2), steroids, and, in those with severe symptoms, epinephrine (intramuscular or subcutaneous).

- *Antihistamine*: Diphenhydramine 50 mg capsules QID × 2–3 days
- Doxepin 25 mg tablets QID × 2–3 days
- Prednisone 10 mg tablets QID × 3 days

Behçet's Disease

- For oral and genital ulcerations, topical steroids or sucralfate solution is first-line therapy for mild isolated ulcerations. Colchicine has also been used to prevent mucocutaneous relapse. For severe mucocutaneous lesions, systemic corticosteroids, azathioprine, pentoxifylline, dapsone, interferon-α, colchicine, and thalidomide have demonstrated benefit.
- Refer to a dermatologist, a rheumatologist, or an ophthalmologist, depending on organ involvement, for ongoing care, which may include systemic immunosuppressive and/or anti-inflammatory drugs.

Candidiasis

The treatments used to manage *Candida* infections vary substantially and are based on the anatomic location of the infection, the patients' underlying disease and immune status, the patients' risk factors for infection, the specific species of *Candida* responsible for infection, and, in some cases, the susceptibility of the *Candida* species to specific antifungal drugs. Identify and correct provocative factors.

- *Topical therapy*:
  Nystatin oral suspension (100,000 units/mL); rinse 5 mL and swallow 4 times/day
  Clotrimazole (Lotrimin) solution 1%; rinse 5 ml and swallow 4 times/day
  Clotrimazole troches (Mycelex) 10 mg; dissolve 1 troche in mouth 5 times/day
  Clotrimazole vaginal tablets 1/2 of 500 mg tablet dissolved in mouth BID
- *Systemic therapy*:
  Fluconazole (Diflucan) 100 mg; 2 tablets on the first day, 1 tablet days 2–7, 1 tablet every other day for days 8–21
  Ketoconazole (Nizoral) 200 mg; 1 tablet everyday with breakfast × 21 days
  Itraconazole (Sporanox) 200 mg; 1 tablet everyday with breakfast × 21 days
  May use shorter duration for less severe infections

Cheilitis Glandularis

- Challenging to treat
- Trials of therapy
- Intralesional corticosteroids as triamcinolone acetonide 5–10 mg/mL; inject 1–3 mL per session with sessions at 3–4 week intervals
- *Systemic antibiotic*: Tetracycline 500 mg TID
- *Systemic corticosteroid*: Prednisone 5 mg tablets #40
  - Take each morning for 8 with breakfast, 8-8-6-6-4-4-2-2 mg, stop
  - Will shorten the course of an individual episode but not change the natural history of the disease

Cheilitis Granulomatosa

The approach to treatment for cheilitis glandularis is based on diagnostic information obtained from histopathologic analysis, the identification of likely etiologic factors responsible for the cheilitis glandularis, and attempts to alleviate or eradicate those causes. It is challenging to treat and needs trials of therapy.

- Intralesional corticosteroids such as triamcinolone acetonide 5–10 mg/mL; inject 1–3 mL per session with sessions at 3–4 week intervals
- *Systemic antibiotic:* Tetracycline 500 mg TID
- *Systemic corticosteroids:* Prednisone 5 mg tablets. Take each morning for 8 days with breakfast, taper the dose and stop. These drugs will shorten the course of an individual episode but not change the natural history of the disease.
- Dapsone 25 mg tablets
  Check baseline complete blood count (CBC), liver function tests, urinalysis, and glucose-6-phosphate red blood cell enzyme level before treatment
- *Systemic therapy:* Prednisone 5 mg tablets. Take each morning with breakfast for 16 days as 8/day × 4 days, 6/day × 4 days, 4/days × 4 days, 2/day × 4 days and stop. This will reduce disease activity as topical corticosteroids or systemic NSAIDs are started.

Erythema Multiforme

Systemic corticosteroid therapy is controversial in erythema multiforme (EM), and some believe it may predispose to complications. Beneficial effects with hemodialysis, plasmapheresis, cyclosporin, immunoglobulin, levamisole, thalidomide, dapsone, and cyclophosphamide have been documented in case reports.

- Topical therapy (compounded rinses)
- *Option 1*: Diphenhydramine 200 mg, viscous lidocaine 90 mL, Maalox suspension 90 mL, distilled water 180 ml. Swish 5 ml for 2 minutes and expectorate 3–4 times/day.
- *Option 2*: Dexamethasone 100 mg, viscous lidocaine 60 ml, diphenhydramine 200 mg, sorbitol 15 ml, Maalox suspension to 275 ml. Swish 5 ml for 2 min and expectorate 3–4 times/day.
- *Systemic therapy*: Prednisone 5 mg tablets. Take each morning with breakfast for 16 days as 8/day × 4 days, 6/day × 4 days, 4/day × 4 days, 2/day × 4 days and then stop. It will reduce disease activity as topical corticosteroids or systemic NSAIDs are started.
  Acyclovir 200 mg tablets (if triggered by herpes simplex virus infection); 1 tablet every 4 hour for 7 days or 1 tablet BID-TID as prophylaxis.

Alternative treatments for erythema multiforme include dapsone, antimalarials, azathioprine, cimetidine, and thalidomide. For ocular involvement, artificial wetting solutions, antibiotic solutions, or ointments may be helpful.

Fissured Tongue

No definitive therapy or medication is required for fissured tongue. If symptomatic, patients with fissured tongue are encouraged to brush the dorsum of the tongue surface 10–15 times with dentifrice after meals and at bedtime to remove debris that causes halitosis.

Geographic Tongue

No medical intervention is required because the lesion is benign and most often asymptomatic. However, Abe et al. report successful treatment with cyclosporin, and Sigal and Mock reported treatment with topical and systemic antihistamines. Topical retinoids and topical corticosteroids are occasionally of benefit. In psoriatic patients, the lesions may resolve during systemic therapy for the psoriasis.

- Brush tongue surface 10–15 times with dentifrice after meals and at bedtime to remove debris that causes halitosis.
- *Topical therapy*:
  Fluocinonide gel/cream 0.05% 60 gm; apply after meals and at bedtime
  Clotrimazole troches (Mycelex) 10 mg; dissolve 1 troche in mouth 5 times/day

Clotrimazole vaginal tablets 1/2 of 500 mg tablet dissolved in mouth BID
Tacrolimus (Protopic) ointment 0.1% 60 gm; apply after meals and at bedtime

Hairy Tongue

The treatment of hairy tongue is variable. In many cases, simply brushing the tongue with a toothbrush or using a commercially available tongue scraper 10–15 times with dentifrice after meals and at bedtime is sufficient to remove elongated filiform papillae and retard the growth of additional ones.

- *Topical therapy*: Dilute H_2O_2 (1 part 3% H_2O_2 : 1 part H_2O); brush tongue after meals and at bedtime for black hairy tongue

Herpangina

Herpangina is a self-limited illness. As such, no specific therapy is indicated. Currently, no antiviral therapy is effective against herpangina. Antibacterial therapy is of no benefit. Recently, considerable efforts have been made in the development of antiviral compounds targeting the capsid protein of enterovirus, as well as viral proteases and proteins involved in enteroviral RNA replication. Treatment is generally supportive and includes the following:

- Hydration
- Antipyretics (e.g. acetaminophen, ibuprofen)
- Topical analgesics (e.g. topical lidocaine)

Herpes Zoster

Episodes of herpes zoster are generally self-limited and resolve without intervention; they tend to be more benign and mild in children than in adults. An enormous number and variety of therapeutic approaches have been proposed over the years, most of which are probably ineffective. Some effective therapies for herpes zoster do exist, however, and these can reduce the extent and duration of symptoms, and possibly the risk of chronic sequelae (e.g. postherpetic neuralgia [PHN]) as well.

- *Topical therapy*:
  Calamine lotion for wet, oozing cutaneous lesions
  Doxepin (Zonalon) cream for pain relief of acute lesions
- *Systemic therapy*:
  Acyclovir 400 mg tablets; 2 tablets 5 times daily × 7–10 days
  Famciclovir 500 mg tablets; 1 tablet 3 times daily × 7 days
  Valacyclovir 500 mg tablets; 2 tablets 3 times daily × 7 days

Lichen Planus

Lichen planus (LP) is a self-limited disease that usually resolves within 8–12 months. Mild cases can be treated with fluorinated topical steroids. More severe cases, especially those with scalp, nail, and mucous membrane involvement, may need more intensive therapy.

- *Topical therapy*:
  Betamethasone cream (0.1%) 60 g; apply after meals and at bedtime
  Fluocinonide gel/cream 0.05% 60 g; apply after meals and at bedtime
  Tacrolimus (Protopic) ointment 0.1% 30 g; apply after meals 3 times daily and at bedtime, do not eat or drink for 30 minutes; taper frequency depending on response
- *Intralesional therapy*: Triamcinolone acetonide 5–10 mg/mL; inject 1–3 mL per session with sessions at 3–4 week intervals
- *Systemic therapy*:
  Prednisone 5 mg tablets. Take each morning with breakfast for 16 days as 8/day × 4 days, 6/day × 4 days, 4/day × 4 days, 2/day × 4 days and then stop. It will reduce disease activity as topical corticosteroids or systemic NSAIDs are started.
  Dapsone 25 mg tablets. Check baseline CBC, liver function tests, urinalysis, and glucose-6-phosphate dehydrogenase enzyme level before treatment. Take each morning with breakfast, 1 × 3 days, 2 × 3 days, 3 × 3 days, 4 × 7 days, and 5 × daily thereafter
  Check CBC and liver function every month for 3 months, then every 3 month thereafter.
  Use for long-term control of disease.
  Hydroxychloroquine (Plaquenil) 250 mg; 2 tablets with breakfast for 4 week, then 1 tablet daily for maintenance.
  Baseline ophthalmology consultation; repeat every 6 month to monitor for retinal toxicity

Lupus Erythematosus

Treatment of systemic lupus erythematosus is guided by the individual patient's manifestations. Fever, rash, musculoskeletal manifestations, and serositis generally respond to treatment with hydroxychloroquine, NSAIDs, and steroids in low-to-moderate doses, as necessary, for acute flares. Medications such as methotrexate may be useful in chronic lupus arthritis, and azathioprine and mycophenolate have been widely used in lupus of moderate severity.

- *Topical therapy*:
  Fluocinonide gel/cream 0.05% 60 g; apply after meals and at bedtime
  Tacrolimus (Protopic) ointment 0.1% 30 g; apply after meals 3 times daily, do not eat or drink for 30 minutes
- *Intralesional therapy*: Triamcinolone acetonide 5–10 mg/mL; inject 1–3 mL per session with sessions at 3-4 week intervals.

Nevus

Medical treatment is typically ineffective and inappropriate for the management of a benign neoplasm such as a melanocytic nevus. All pigmented nevi should be excised, if reasonable from a surgical point of view.

Pemphigoid

As in other autoimmune bullous diseases, the goal of therapy is to decrease blister formation, to promote healing of blisters and erosions, and to determine the minimal dose of medication necessary to control the disease process. Therapy must be individualized for each patient, keeping in mind pre-existing conditions and other patient-specific factors.

- Refer to a dermatologist or an ophthalmologist, depending on organ involvement, for ongoing care, which may include systemic immunosuppressive and/or anti-inflammatory drugs.
- *For localized oral pemphigoid/gingival pemphigoid, apply topical therapy*: Fluocinonide 0.05% gel/cream 60 g. Apply to early lesions after meals and at bedtime. Do not apply to ulcers.
  May be used for 1–2 hours with mouthguard for occlusive therapy
- *Systemic therapy for severe, chronic disease*:
  Prednisone 5 mg tablets. Take each morning with breakfast for 16 days as 8/day × 4 days, 6/day × 4 days, 4/day × 4 days, 2/day × 4 days and then stop. It will reduce disease activity as topical corticosteroids or systemic NSAIDs are started.
  Dapsone 25 mg tablets. Check baseline CBC, liver function tests, urinalysis, and glucose-6-phosphate dehydrogenase enzyme level before treatment. Take each morning with breakfast, 1 × 3 days, 2 × 3 days, 3 × 3 days, 4 × 7 days, and 5 × daily thereafter,
  Check CBC and liver function every month for 3 months, then every 3 month thereafter.
  Use for long-term control of disease.
  Tetracycline and niacinamide: 500 mg of each administered TID. Use for long-term control of disease.

Pemphigus Vulgaris

The aim of treatment in pemphigus vulgaris is the same as in other autoimmune bullous diseases, which is to decrease blister formation, promote healing of blisters and erosions, and determine the minimal dose of medication necessary to control the disease process. Coordinate overall management with patient's internist/primary care physician since treatment of this disease requires systemic immunosuppression and/or use of anti-inflammatory drugs.

Management of oral lesions will consist of systemic immunosuppressive agents. Local/intralesional therapy may be a useful adjunct following an initial good measurable response to systemic glucocorticosteroid dosing.

- *Systemic therapy:* Prednisone 10 mg tablets. Take each morning with breakfast at a total daily dose of 1 mg/kg of body weight. Taper slowly over several months as clinical response permits to maintenance dosing. Management of prednisone side effects is important.
- *Corticosteroid-sparing systemic therapy*:
  Azathioprine 1–3 mg/kg; dosing spaced morning and evening
  Mycophenolate mofetil 500 mg tablets; 1.5 gm BID

- *Severe or unresponsive disease*:
  Plasmapheresis
  Pulse cyclophosphamide (Cytoxan) IV for 3 week Monitor response. Continue on orally administered immunosuppressants.
  IVIg therapy
- *Local therapy for focal residual lesions*: intralesional triamcinolone suspension 10 mg/mL.

Plasma Cell Gingivitis

Identify contact allergen(s) and avoid exposure.
- *Topical therapy:* Fluocinonide gel/cream 0.05% 60 gm; apply after meals and at bedtime
- *Systemic therapy:* Griseofulvin 250 mg tablets; take 1 with each meal for 7 week

Radiation-induced Mucositis

- *Topical therapy*:
  Benzydamine rinses
  Saline/bicarbonate rinses 2.5 mL each in 125 mL water; 5 mL rinsed bid
  Chlorhexidine 0.12% compounded as alcohol-free formula
  Store in a light-protective container. 15-30 ml rinse BID
- *Systemic therapy*: Analgesics

Recurrent Aphthous Stomatitis

Identify and correct predisposing factors for recurrent aphthous stomatitis (RAS). Ensure that patients brush atraumatically (e.g. with a small-headed, soft toothbrush) and avoid eating particularly hard or sharp foods (e.g. toast, potato crisps) and avoid other trauma to the oral mucosa. Classify disease into simple versus complex.

Simple Aphthosis

- Amlexanox paste 5 gm (Aphthasol); apply to ulcers after meals and at bedtime
- Fluocinonide 0.05% gel/cream 60 gm. Apply to early lesions after meals and at bedtime. Do not apply to ulcers.
- *Compounded rinse option 1*: Diphenhydramine parenteral (or 12.5 mg/5 mL non-alcoholic elixer) 200 mg, viscous lidocaine 90 mL, Maalox suspension 90 mL, distilled water 180 mL, Rinse 5 mL-expectorate 4–6 times daily.
- *Compounded rinse option 2*: Dexamethasone (10 mg/mL) 10 mL, diphenhydramine 200 mg, viscous lidocaine 60 mL, Maalox suspension 85–275 mL, Rinse 5 mL—expectorate 3–5 times daily.

Complex Aphthosis

Laboratory evaluation for correctable causes: CBC, red blood cell folate, serum ferritin, serum vitamin B_{12}, serum iron studies, serum zinc.

- Topical therapy as for simple aphthosis
- Systemic therapy for severe, painful, chronic complex aphthosis
  Prednisone 5 mg tablets. Take each morning with breakfast for 8 days with dose tapering and stop. This will shorten the course of an individual episode but not change the natural history of the disease.
  Colchicine 0.5 mg tablets. Take 1 each morning with breakfast for 1 week; if tolerated, increase to 2 tablets each morning. May suppress disease activity.
  Pentoxifylline (Trental) 400 mg tablets; 1 tablet 3 times/day with meals
  Dapsone 25 mg tablets. Check baseline CBC, liver function tests, urinalysis and glucose-6-phosphate dehydrogenase enzyme level before treatment. Take each morning with breakfast, 1 × 3 days, 2 × 3 days, 3 × 3 days, 4 × 7 days, and 5 × daily thereafter.
  Check CBC and liver function every month for 3 month, then every 3 month thereafter. Use for long-term control of disease.

Recurrent Herpes Simplex Labialis or Stomatitis

- *Topical therapy*:
  Penciclovir cream (Denavir) 1% 1.5 gm tube; apply at the onset of symptoms every 2 hour × 4 days
  Docosanol cream (Abreva) 10%; apply topically at the onset of symptoms 2–3 hour 5 times daily
  Acyclovir ointment 5% 3 gm tube; apply at the onset of symptoms 6 times daily × 7 days
- *Systemic therapy*:
  Acyclovir 200 mg tablets, 1 tablet 5 times daily × 7 days. Start medication with premonitory symptoms to shorten the course of the episode.
  Acyclovir 200 mg tablets, 3 tablets daily to prevent reactivation in bone marrow transplant recipients.

Sjögren's Syndrome

Many people can manage the dry eyes and dry mouth associated with Sjögren's syndrome by using over-the-counter eyedrops and sipping water more frequently. But some people may need prescription medications, or even surgery. To relieve dry eyes, consider undergoing a minor surgical procedure to seal the tear ducts that drain tears from eyes (punctal occlusion). Collagen or silicone plugs are inserted into the ducts for a temporary closure. Collagen plugs eventually dissolve, but silicone plugs stay in place until they fall out or are removed.

- *Topical therapy*:
  Moisten mouth with cool water or ice-chips
  Avoid alcohol-containing mouth rinses
  Avoid drugs that produce xerostomia
  Limit caffeine intake

Use vaseline on lips at night (a thin coating)
Drink milk with meals
Saliva substitutes: Liquid, tablet, or gel forms. Available over the counter

- *Systemic therapy*:
  Pilocarpine (Salagen) 5 mg tablets; take 1 tablet 3 times daily
  Cevimeline capsules (Evoxac) 30 mg capsules; take 1 capsule 3 times daily.

Stevens-Johnson Syndrome

- *Topical therapy (compounded rinses)*:
  Option 1: Diphenhydramine 200 mg, viscous lidocaine 90 mL, Maalox suspension 90 mL, distilled water 180 mL. Swish 5 ml for 2 minutes and expectorate 3–4 times/day.
  Option 2: Dexamethasone 100 mg, viscous lidocaine 60 mL, diphenhydramine 200 mg, sorbitol 15 mL, Maalox suspension to 275 mL. Swish 5 mL for 2 min and expectorate 3–4 times/day
- *Systemic therapy*:
  Prednisone 5 mg tablets. Take each morning with breakfast for 16 days as 8/day × 4 days, 6/day × 4 days, 4/day × 4 days, 2/day × 4 days and then stop. It will reduce disease activity as topical corticosteroids or systemic NSAIDs are started.
  Acyclovir 200 mg tablets (if triggered by herpes simplex virus infection); 1 tablet every 4 hour for 7 days or 1 tablet BID-TID as prophylaxis.

Tuberculosis

Isolate patients with possible tuberculosis infection in a private room with negative pressure (air exhausted to outside or through a high-efficiency particulate air filter). Staff must wear high-efficiency disposable masks sufficient to filter the tubercle bacillus. Continue isolation until sputum smears are negative for 3 consecutive determinations (usually after approximately 2–4 weeks of treatment). For initial empirical treatment of TB, start patients on a 4-drug regimen: isoniazid, rifampin, pyrazinamide, and either ethambutol or streptomycin.

- *Systemic therapy (prolonged treatment with at least 2 drugs)*:
  Isoniazid 300 mg daily × 6 months
  Rifampin 450–600 mg daily × 6 months
  Ethambutol 15 mg/kg daily for first 2 months
  Pyrazinamide 1.5–2.5 mg/kg for first 2 months

Once the TB isolate is known to be fully susceptible, ethambutol (or streptomycin, if it is used as a fourth drug) can be discontinued.

Wegener's Granulomatosis

- *Systemic therapy*:
  Sulfamethoxazole/trimethoprim (Bactrim DS) Septra DS: 1 twice daily
  Prednisone 1 mg/kg daily
  Cyclophosphamide

Complementary and Alternative Medicine Techniques Available for Dentistry

There are five general categories of complementary and alternative medicine (CAM):

1. Alternative medical systems
2. Mind-body interventions
3. Biologically based therapy
4. Manipulative and body based methods
5. Energy therapy.

Alternative medical systems are based on theory and practice separate from allopathic medicine. These systems include homeopathy, naturopathy, *Ayurveda*, Chinese medicine and chiropractic manipulation.

Homeopathy

It is a set of procedures using highly diluted medications made from animal, mineral and vegetable sources. These are used as substitutes for antibiotics and pain medication. This methodology incorporates the use of small quantities of medicaments to cause symptoms the patient is experiencing. It is a natural system of medicine that stimulates the body to heal on its own. A homeopathic dose of Arnica in dentistry is thought to speed the healing, whereas Hypericum is useful in desensitizing a tooth.

Naturopathy

Naturopathy is an alternative medical system based on therapies of nutrition, medicinal plants, dietary supplements, natural foods, light, warmth, massage, fresh air, regular exercise and the avoidance of medications.

Dietary supplements are products (other than tobacco) taken by mouth that may include vitamins, minerals, herbs, botanicals, amino acids, enzymes, organ tissues (glandular products) and metabolites. They are considered foods, not drugs, and are regulated by the Food and Drug Administration (FDA).

Ayurveda

Ayurveda (meaning "science of life") is an alternative medical system that emphasizes body, mind and spirit remedies. Diet, exercise (*Yoga*), meditation, herbs, massage, exposure to sunlight and controlled breathing are used to treat and prevent disease. Ayurvedic medicine strives to restore the harmony of the individual. Yoga is a discipline that focuses on the body's musculature, posture, breathing and consciousness.

Traditional Chinese Medicine

Traditional Chinese medicine is the ancient system of healthcare from China-based on the concept of qi (pronounced "chee") energy that flows through the body. Disease occurs when qi is disrupted, causing a yin and yang imbalance.

Therapies include herbal/nutritional remedies, physical exercise, meditation, acupuncture and curing massage. Qi Gong (pronounced "chee gung") is a practice that combines movement, meditation, and breathing to improve qi, circulation and immune function. Ginseng is a botanical dietary supplement thought to improve heart function, work as an aphrodisiac and stimulant.

Acupuncture

Acupuncture involves placing fine needles into acupuncture points. It is divided into several treatment modalities, which have an indirect influence on the endocrine and reticular formation of the brainstem. The theory behind this therapy is that the body is made of 14 main channels that contain 700–800 acupuncture points. Energy flow from organ to organ is through these channels. Nerves can be stimulated or sedated by the placement of needles into acupuncture points. The indications for acupuncture are anesthesia allergies, acute abscess or cellulitis, patient preference, or other respiratory disease, sinus problems, cold symptoms, or as a supplement to LA or GA. Acupuncture is contraindicated in dermatitis, hemophilia, pregnancy, uncooperative patients, patients that may make sudden or uncontrolled movements, exhausted, fasting, emotionally upset or perspiring patients.

Mind-Body Interventions

Mind-Body Interventions are based on the theory and practice of enhancing the mind to affect body functions and disease symptoms. They include prayer, meditation, mental healing, and creative outlets such as art, music or dance. The most frequently used complementary and alternative medicine (CAM) therapy is prayer. Religious prayers are well documented for use in healing and spiritual insight.

Dental practitioners may use imagery, relaxation, rehearsals, biofeedback, hypnosis, and paranormal health remedies as complementary or alternative techniques for conventional dental treatment. Many of these, nontraditional therapies are recommended for the dental phobic patients, who have an irrational fear of dentistry. Reasons for dental anxiety can be from direct experience or indirect experience. Whatever the reason, affected people will avoid dental visit and self treat their chronic pain. These patients will seek dental care when they can no longer tolerate the pain. Assessing such patients is the first step in building a working relationship. Increase the level of attention to the patient's verbal and nonverbal communication. Use visual, auditory or kinesthetic modes of communication, according to patient's ease of understanding, to reassure the patient and help establish rapport. When you use predictable behavior, explain procedures, and give encouragement and reinforcement, the patients feel a sense of control and know they can stop any treatment at any time. Some dental phobic people require seeing a psychologist first. When the patient is ready to see the dentist, an initial oral examination is scheduled. After the patient is treatment planned, coping mechanisms are incorporated into their psychological visits.

Imagery, Relaxation and Rehearsals

Desensitization is the most common approach to treating the dental phobic, using relaxation and imagery to calm the anxious or fearful patient. Relaxation techniques and visual imagery techniques are often practiced together. Controlled breathing is a technique of relaxation. Rehearsals are another technique of desensitization in which the patient is placed in a situation and is able to control the stimuli which lets the patient feel a sense of control in the situation. The patient and therapist spend long periods of time becoming accustomed to a source of anxiety and practice the event, such as an anesthesia injection.

Biofeedback

Biofeedback is a behavioral science in which humans learn to develop conscious control or change internal body processes using imagery and relaxation techniques. People calm down when a stressful event is over or when they have done something to cope with it. When the body is repeatedly aroused, one or more functions may become permanently overactive and damage to body tissues results. Biofeedback changes habitual reactions to stress that can cause pain or disease. Measurements of how physical processes react to stress are used to teach the patient how their bodies react. Biofeedback is used to improve the body's immune system for healing, for the treatment of the dental phobic patient and the patient with temporomandibular joint disorder (TMD). Not all people respond to hypnosis, but biofeedback can be used for everybody.

Hypnosis

Hypnosis is a technique that uses a natural altered state of consciousness. The hypnotic state is a deeply relaxed state that is similar to the experience felt prior to falling asleep. A determination is made as to whether the patient is suggestible for hypnotic induction. Once the patient is tested on how receptive they will be, the next step is to induce hypnosis using verbal suggestions or eye fixation. Once the hypnotic state is entered, physiologic changes occur in the patient. After the operative procedure, the patient is dehypnotized.

Paranormal Health Remedies

Paranormal health remedies and divinations are less frequently used Mind-Body Interventions. They include past life regression and divinations. Divination means predicting the future or any outcome using a specific course of action. It includes reading astrological charts, numerology, I Ching readings, Fortune tellers, Tarot cards or tea leaves.

Biologically Based Therapy

Biologically based therapy is the theory and practice of using substances found in nature. Practitioners use herbs, foods, dietary supplements, aromatherapy and specific regimens to treat or prevent disease. They have become the CAM technique most frequently used after prayer. Dental mouth rinses containing various herbal essences are thought to help prevent periodontal problems. Herbs with medicinal properties are a useful and effective source of treatment for various disease processes. Dietary supplements in the form of antioxidant vitamins C and E are recommended for gingival inflammation. Dietary supplements of the mineral magnesium citrate are recommended to improve muscle function in an individual with a high-fat, high protein diet.

The below mentioned herbs are commonly used for dental problems.

Alfalfa: The leaves, petals, flowers, and sprouts are commonly used to treat stomach and blood disorders. One of the richest sources of trace minerals and an antioxidant, alfalfa is high in calcium, iron, magnesium, phosphorus, potassium, chlorine, and vitamin K. Alfalfa is useful in cases of hemorrhaging and fungal infections and is an excellent choice as a mineral supplement.

Aloe Vera: The aloe vera plant is an ingredient in many cosmetics because it heals moisturizes, and softens skin. Applied externally, aloe vera gel is excellent for soothing inflamed gums and sores in the mouth. Aloe vera gel should not be taken internally in large quantities by those who have hemorrhoids or an irritated colon and by pregnant women.

Anise: Also known as sweet fennel, its seeds are used in medicine and as a flavoring. An anti-inflammatory herb, anise is commonly used in tea form to soothe the gums. Fennel seeds whole can be chewed to eliminate bad breath.

Bee Pollen: Fresh pollen obtained from bees contains amino acids, various minerals, vitamins, and other chemicals and nutrients. It is effective for combating fatigue, depression, and colon disorders. Pollen has an antimicrobial effect. A small percentage of the population is allergic to bee pollen. Use with caution, starting with small amounts and discontinuing, if a rash, wheezing, or other symptoms develop.

Chamomile: Commonly used as a nerve tonic, sleep aid, and digestive aid, chamomile is also a homeopathic remedy. It can be used for pain and swelling or can be taken as a hot tea to promote relaxation or as a mouthwash to soothe inflamed, irritated gums.

Chickweed: Its leaves are used to soothe skin irritations. Chickweed mouthwash soothes inflamed, irritated mouth tissues associated with oral cancer; it also helps to relieve pain from canker sores and other mouth sores.

Cloves: They have antiseptic, stimulant, and antiemetic (vomiting preventive) properties and are used to treat the mouth, stomach, intestines, circulation, and lungs. Oil of cloves can be rubbed on sore gums and teeth to ease pain or can be chewed whole to diminish bad breath.

Eucalyptus: It yields a powerfully antiseptic essential oil that has long been used medicinally. As its leaves have commonly been used to lower fevers, the eucalyptus is sometimes known as the "fever tree." Rub eucalyptus oil on sore, inflamed gums for temporary relief.

Evening Primrose: Its oil is used to treat skin disorders, arthritis, alcoholism, and other disorders. It also aids in weight loss and in reducing high blood pressure. Rubbing the oil on sore, inflamed gums provides temporary relief.

Garlic: It is used as a natural antibiotic that is good for fighting infections caused by fungi or bacteria. It helps strengthen the immune system and is used to lower blood pressure. Garlic is also used to treat arteriosclerosis, asthma, arthritis, and digestive and circulatory problems. Fresh oil of garlic or raw cloves is considered the most effective forms.

Marigold: Commonly used as a homeopathic remedy marigold flowers have been used internally as a diuretic, a stimulant, and an antispasmodic. Externally, they are used in the treatment of burns, wounds, and impetigo of the scalp. It can be used as a mouthwash to help relieve ulcers, wounds, or inflamed areas, and to relax muscles associated with tension in the jaw joint and pressure from braces.

Parsley: Chewing on a sprig of sweet, aromatic parsley will help eliminate bad breath.

Peppermint: It has been used to treat the stomach, intestines, and muscles, and to improve circulation. The leaves and flowering tops are now used to treat colic, fever, convulsions, and especially nausea and diarrhea. Use peppermint oil for toothache. Soak a cotton ball in the oil and place it in the cavity or rub it on the tooth. It can also be used as a mouthwash to relieve gum inflammation.

Red Clover: Used mainly as a blood purifier, it is also helpful in treating acne, boils, and skin infections. It is also effective as a mild sedative. For a general calming effect, drink warm red clover tea. Red clover mouthwash is healing for irritated, diseased gums. After making red clover tea, prepare an ointment from the strained blossoms and leaves and rub on gums that are abscessed from disease, or sore and inflamed from root canal therapy or other dental procedures.

Shepherd's Purse: The tops are used for their astringent, diuretic, and stimulant properties. Use the fresh tops of shepherd's purse to help stop bleeding after tooth extraction.

Tea Tree Oil: It is used in several commercial products including mouthwash and toothpaste. It is highly antiseptic and antifungal for cuts and abrasions, as well as warts and cold sores. Rub tea tree oil directly on sore, inflamed gums for temporary relief.

Thyme: It is a powerful antiseptic (bacilli exposed to thyme essence do not survive for more than forty minutes), and the leaves and flowers are used to treat chronic respiratory problems, colds, sore throats, and the flu. Use a salve made of thyme, myrrh, and golden-seal to treat oral herpes. As thyme is a uterine stimulant, therapeutic doses in any form should be avoided by pregnant women.

Nutrition

Nutritional diets are thought to prevent or control illness and to promote health and wellness. Orthomolecular therapies treat disease with varying concentrations of chemicals. Dentists may work with a nutritionist to test and balance body chemistry by analyzing hormones, enzymes, digestion, assimilation, vitamins, minerals, carbohydrates, fats, proteins, and other body constituents. Dentists will use dental materials they believe have few side effects. While amalgam restorations and nickel containing crowns are traditional dentistry, dentists may choose ceramic, porcelain, gold, or composite dental materials.

Biological Therapy

Biological therapies such as the use of laetrile and shark cartilage are used to treat cancer. Bee pollen is used to treat autoimmune and inflammatory diseases.

Aromatherapy

Aromatherapy is the inhalation or application on the skin of essential oils to promote healing and wellness. Low doses of essential oils are believed to be the safest when diluted in carrier oil. Diluted oils are massaged directly over the area that needs treatment. Application by inhalation or bath is also appropriate for essential oil therapy. They can be used in combination with herbs, to be more effective. Essential oils kill pathogenic bacteria by disrupting their life cycle, leaving beneficial bacteria intact. Bacteria typically do not acquire a resistance to essential oils similar to antibiotic resistance. Essential oils act quickly in the body, some are detectable on the breath within minutes, and are eliminated from the body within several hours. Repeated applications may be required, especially when treating acute disorders. Too much essential oil may cause adverse reactions. The amount of Lavender for sedating is in low dilution, whereas high dilution is stimulating. Body massage oils are blended with a saturated oil. The more saturated the oil, the thicker it becomes, causing it to stay longer on the skin. Vegetable oils high in vitamins A, E and F are soothing, contain nutrients that enrich the skin and are among the best carrier oil for essential oils.

Manipulative and Body Based Methods

These methods use the theory and practice of manipulation and/or movement of the body. Dentists may incorporate the use of physical therapy, chiropractic or massage therapies for relief of facial pain, correction of jaw malalignment, muscle tightness and spasm, and TMD because muscular involvement is a major component of the disorder. **Table 1** outlines the physical therapy treatment regimens used in dentistry.

Table 1: Dental physical therapy treatment

Therapy	*Regimens*
Acustimulation	Low frequency electrical stimulation of areas to increase the body's production of endorphins.
Electrical stimulation	High frequency electrical stimulation of muscles produce muscle contractions, which increase circulation and decrease pain.
HENE laser	Low intensity laser used to decrease muscle spasms. control pain and exert anti-inflammatory effects.
Ice therapy	Cold icepack treatment of muscles to reduce pain and swelling.
Iontophoresis	Electrical source used to facilitate medication penetration into the tissues.
Massage therapy	Rubbing of muscles to increase circulation and relaxation, and decrease muscle spasm.
Medcosonolator	A device used to produce ultrasonic and electrical stimulation.
Moist heat	Therapy moist, hot towels used to increase circulation and relaxation, and decrease muscle spasm.
Motor point electrical stimulation	Technique used to increase circulation to damaged nerves and to stimulate muscles.
Phonophoresis	Hydrocortisone ointment forced through the skin with ultrasonic sound waves to a depth of 5 cm to reduce Inflammation.
Transcutaneous electrical nerve stimulator (TENS)	Electrical device used to decrease pain by transferring energy through the nervous system and increase endorphin production.
Ultrasound	High frequency sound waves produce a deep heating effect that increases muscle relaxation and resorption of adhesions and calcification deposits
Vasocoolant spray and stretch	Fluoromethane or ethyl chloride spray used to decrease pain and muscle spasm. Used in conjunction with gentle muscle massage to stretch painful muscles

Chiropractic Manipulation

It is the theory and manipulation of the hard tissue structures of the body. Skeletal adjustments are made to correct the vertebral alignment of the spine to restore normal brain and nerve transmission and help recovery from illness. The chiropractic diagnosis consists of taking an accurate medical history, an examination focused on detecting muscle strength versus weakness and the range of motion of the spine. Radiographs are exposed to identify misalignments of the vertebral column and areas of spinal stress.

Massage

Massage is the manipulation of the soft tissues of the human body.

Energy Therapy

Energy therapy is the theory and practice of manipulating biofields and bioelectromagnetic fields to affect energy. The application of pressure and/or manipulating the body by placing the hands in or through biofields is thought to improve circulation, immune function, and healing. A common biofield therapy is therapeutic touch that involves passing the clinician's hands over the patient to promote healing. The use of pulsed, alternating or direct current, and magnetic fields treats asthma, cancer, manages pain, or migraine headaches through bioelectromagnetic fields.

Complementary and alternative medicine in dentistry includes various treatment modalities. Many procedures are under scientific investigation to determine effectiveness. Dental patients request CAM therapy in an attempt to save money and to prevent invasive procedures. Scientific verification of efficacy of CAM procedures are required to enable using these in standard practice.

8

Guidelines for Management of Medically Compromised Patients in Dental Office

It is the management of patients in whom the dental treatment may need modification according to their medical condition. The goal of identifying such patients is to evaluate any source of infection that may compromise successful medical or surgical therapy and restore optimal oral health and function. The screening of the patients can be done by:

- Full mouth intraoral radiographs along with panoramic radiograph (if dentulous)
- Panoramic radiograph only if edentulous or not able to take intraoral films
- Thorough medical and dental history, including medications documented on our own
- Complete dental charting, periodontal charting if appropriate, but periodontal probing of all teeth will routinely be accomplished.
- Physician consultation to corroborate medical history and coordinate dental and medical care.
- Initiate preventive therapy.

The following patients might require antibiotic premedication before initiating a dental procedure:

- Prosthetic heart valves
- Patients with congenital heart disease
- Heart murmurs, e.g. MVP (with incompetence) and history of rheumatic heart disease
- Poorly controlled diabetic patients
- Dialysis patients, those with AV shunts and those on peritoneal dialysis
- Organ transplant patients, pre- and post-transplant
- Artificial joint replacement patients
- Radiation therapy patients, depending on procedure
- Chemotherapy patients, including bone marrow transplant
- Down syndrome patients (many have cardiac defects)
- Immunocompromised patients (depending on treatment)

The following pages highlight the most common medical conditions that may be encountered by the dental staff and their possible management.

- A few of the following steps prior to the treatment of such patients will aid in their preoperative management:

- A good and detailed medical history of the patient should be recorded and updated during each subsequent visit.
- The medical condition should be mentioned in the consent form.
- Any previous unpleasant dental experience should be reported.
- Previous hospitalization of the patient and the reason for it should be recorded.
- Prefer early morning appointments except in cardiac patients, which are preferred in late morning.
- In school oral health program, treat severe medically compromised patients at the program centers.

Cardiac Problems

Patients should be instructed always to maintain good oral hygiene. Effective painless LA is essential, and an aspirating syringe should be used. Epinephrine-containing LA should not be given in excessive doses to patient taking beta-blockers, which may induce hypertension and cardiovascular complications. Vital signs and vital organ status should be evaluated prior to deciding on the LA in hypertensive patients. If the vital organ status is normal, then the type of LA is decided by the blood pressure levels. Lidocaine with epinephrine may be used in well-controlled patients. Epinephrine is contraindicated in patients with ≥160 mm Hg systolic blood pressure. Use prilocaine or bupivacaine in mild hypertensives and mepivacaine with epinephrine in moderate hypertensives. Dental treatment is deferred in severe hypertension patients with ≥180 mm Hg systolic blood pressure.

Dental treatment must be delayed for 6 months following a massive MI and for 3 months with a minor MI. Use mepivacaine without epinephrine for the first 6 months of dental treatment and then evaluate, if LA with epinephrine can be given. Following recovery, if the patient is on digitalis then epinephrine is contraindicated, along with other drugs such as macrolides, tetracycline, aspirin and NSAIDs. These drugs cause digitalis toxicity.

Assure the patient. Stress free short, late morning appointments are recommended. Antibiotic prophylaxis is recommended for cardiac patients to prevent infective endocarditis. It is given according to the recommendation of the cardiologist in the situations mentioned in **Tables 1 and 2**. The antibiotic prophylaxis regimen that needs to be administered to the patients prior to the dental procedures is mentioned in **Table 3**.

Diabetes Mellitus

A carefully constructed questionnaire can give some indications that a patient could be at risk of being diabetic or be an undiagnosed diabetic, especially type 2. The classical symptoms of diabetes mellitus (DM) include: Polydypsia, polyuria and polyphagia. The findings such as recent weight loss, irritability, dry mouth, frequent infections and history of poor wound healing are also indicative of possible diabetes. It is recommended that a patient suspected

Table 1: Cardiac conditions for which prophylaxis is or is not recommended

Endocarditis Prophylaxis Recommended
High-risk category • Prosthetic cardiac valves including bioprosthetic and homograft valves • Previous bacterial endocarditis • Complex cyanotic congenital heart disease (e.g. single ventricle states, transposition of the great arteries and tetralogy of Fallot) • Surgically constructed systemic—pulmonary shunts
Moderate risk category • Most other congenital cardiac malformations (other than above and below) • Acquired valvular dysfunction (e.g. rheumatic heart disease) • Hypertrophic cardiomyopathy • Mitral valve prolapse with valvular regurgitation and/or thickened leaflets
Endocarditis Prophylaxis not Recommended
Negligible risk category • Isolated secundum atrial septal defect • Surgical repair of atrial septal defect, ventricular septal defect, or patent ductus arteriosus • Previous coronary artery bypass graft surgery • Mitral valve prolapse without valvular regurgitation • Previous Kawasaki's disease without valvular dysfunction • Previous rheumatic fever without valvular dysfunction • Physiologic, functional, or innocent heart murmurs • Cardiac pacemakers (intravascular and epicardial) and implanted defibrillators

by the dentist to be diabetic, should be referred to a physician for proper evaluation and diagnosis.

Properly controlled type 1 and type 2 diabetic patients usually can undergo all dental treatments without the need for any special precautions. The dentist must know the type and dose of insulin as well as any other medications that the patient is currently taking. Consultation with the patient's physician is a must when:

- The patient has systemic complications of diabetes such as heart or renal disease.
- The patient has difficulty to control diabetes or is under high insulin dosage.
- The patient has an acute oral infection such as periapical or periodontal abscess.

The main hazard during dental care is hypoglycemia, as dental treatment may disrupt the normal pattern of food intake. Blood sugar level (Glucometer) should be checked and controlled. Early morning appointments are preferred which will minimize the risk of stress-induced hypoglycemia. The appointments should be scheduled before or after periods of peak insulin activity. LA can usually be safely used. The epinephrine level in LA has no significant effect

Table 2: Dental procedures for which prophylaxis is or is not recommended

Endocarditis Prophylaxis Recommended

- Dental extractions
- Periodontal procedures including surgery, scaling and root planing, probing, recall maintenance
- Dental implant placement and reimplantation of avulsed tooth
- Endodontic instrumentation or surgery only beyond the apex
- Subgingival placement of antibiotic fibers/strips
- Initial placement of orthodontic bands but not brackets
- Intraligamentary local anesthetic injections
- Prophylactic cleaning of teeth or implants where bleeding is anticipated

Endocarditis Prophylaxis not Recommended

- Restorative dentistry procedures with/without retraction cord
- Local anesthetic injections (non-intraligamentary)
- Intracanal endodontic treatment; post-placement and build-up
- Placement of rubber dams
- Postoperative suture removal
- Placement of removable prosthodontic/orthodontic appliances
- Electrosurgery after postoperative suture removal
- Taking of oral impressions
- Fluoride treatments
- Taking of oral radiographs
- Orthodontic appliance adjustment
- Shedding of primary teeth

Table 3: Suggested antibiotic prophylaxis regimens for a dental procedure

	Drug	*Regimen: Single dose 30–60 minutes before procedure*	
		Adults	*Children*
Oral	Amoxicillin	2 g	50 mg/kg
Unable to take orally	Ampicillin or	2 g IM or IV	50 mg/kg IM or IV
	Cefazolin or Ceftriaxone	1 g IM or IV	50 mg/kg IM or IV
Allergic to penicillin or ampicillin (Oral)	Cephalexin or	2 g	50 mg/kg
	Clindamycin or	600 mg	20 mg/kg
	Azithromycin or Clarithromycin	500 mg	15 mg/kg
Allergic to penicillin or ampicillin and unable to take orally	Cefazolin or Ceftriaxone	1 gm IM or IV	50 mg/kg IM or IV
	or Clindamycin	600 mg IM or IV	20 mg/kg IM or IV

on blood sugar. Drugs that can disturb diabetic control (aspirin and steroids) must be avoided.

Routine dental treatment or short minor surgery under LA can be carried out with no special precautions apart from ensuring that it does not interfere with eating. It is absolutely critical that the patients eat their normal meal before dental treatment. Taking insulin without eating is the primary cause of hypoglycemia. If the patient is restricted from eating before treatment (e.g. for conscious sedation), normal insulin doses will need to be reduced to half of regular insulin and no NPH insulin. Type II patients should skip oral hypoglycemic agents for that day. If the patient is allowed to eat before the treatment, normal insulin doses should be taken, but NPH dose should be reduced to half. Type II patients may continue with regular oral hypoglycemic agents. Orofacial infections should be treated immediately by antibiotics and appropriate incision and drainage, if needed.

Anemia

Deficiency Anemia

Anemia is a decrease in the level of circulating hemoglobin below the normal reference range for a patient's age and sex. It can be caused by lack of iron, vitamin B_{12} or folate. The different deficiencies produce different effects on the erythrocyte. Iron deficiency produces small cells and lack of vitamin B_{12} or folate results in large erythrocytes.

Deficiency states are corrected by replacement therapy. Iron deficiency may be due to dietary factors or due to loss of blood. Vitamin B_{12} deficiency, known as pernicious anemia, is not due to dietary problems but is caused by poor absorption of the vitamin. This is a result of defective intrinsic factor function caused by autoantibody attack.

Pernicious anemia is of interest to dentists as it is one of the complications of nitrous oxide abuse. The dentist should be aware of the cause and the extent of the patient's anemia. Local Anesthesia (LA) is satisfactory for pain control. Oral manifestations of anemia include angular stomatitis, atrophic glossitis and soreness of the tongue. Candidiasis can be aggravated by anemia and may be the presenting feature. Paterson-Kelly (Plummer-Vinson) syndrome of glossitis and dysphagia is uncommon.

Aspirin and NSAIDs should not be administered, as they cause platelet dysfunction, gastritis and acidosis. Among the antibiotics, penicillin, clindamycin and cephalosporins are safe to administer in anemic patients, but macrolides should be given with caution in iron deficiency anemia.

In severe cases of anemia, dental treatment is deferred until the patient is stabilized. In moderate cases, use bupivacaine with 1:200,000 epinephrine for major procedures and mepivacaine without epinephrine for minor procedures.

Hemolytic Anemia

Hemolytic anemia can be the result of extrinsic factors (e.g. malaria) or problems with hemoglobin. Included among the conditions that produce defects in hemoglobin are sickle cell disease, thalassemia and glucose 6-phosphate dehydrogenase deficiency.

Oral manifestations include painful infarcts in the jaws; pulpal symptoms are common in the absence of any obvious dental disease, and hair-on-end appearance on lateral skull X-ray in sickle cell disease. Enlargement of the maxilla is seen in thalassemia major due to bone marrow expansion.

Drugs that can potentially cause hemolysis such as Aspirin and NSAIDs should be stopped. Avoid acetoaminophen and codeine sulphate in G_6PD deficiency anemia. Instead use codeine phosphate and meperidine in these patients. Penicillin V or clindamycin should be given as prophylactic antibiotics for surgical procedures, and infections must be treated vigorously, as the patient may be immunocompromised, in cases where the spleen is non-functional or has been removed.

Local anesthesia (LA) is the safest method for pain control. It is preferred to avoid prilocain which (in over dose) may precipitate methemoglobinemia. Hepatitis B or C or HIV carriage may be a complication in repeatedly transfused patients.

Bleeding Disorders

The family history should be well recorded to determine whether the bleeding disorder is inherited or an acquired problem. Medical report and consultation with the hematologist may be required for patients on anticoagulant treatment. No surgical procedure, no matter how minor, should be performed on a patient with a bleeding disorder without prior consultation with the patient's hematologist or physician.

Some bleeding parameters can change frequently, therefore laboratory tests are needed within a week or closer to the time of dental treatment. Dental procedures should be limited according to the medical condition. It is safe to continue with minor dental procedures, if the platelet counts are >50,000/mm^3. For outpatient periodontal or oral surgical procedures, the platelet count should be >75,000/mm^3 and it should be >100,000/mm^3 for major surgical procedures. Platelet transfusion may be required before surgery.

Avoid aspirin and NSAIDs in patient with bleeding tendency (e.g. hemophilia). Avoid erythromycin and ketoconazol in patients taking warfarin (inhibits warfarin metabolism). Always obtain a PT from the physician prior to probing a patient on Coumadin. The physician should be consulted about discontinuing or reducing anticoagulant dosage until the desired INR is achieved. Most clinicians nowadays do not recommend discontinuing anticoagulation for many procedures, as this has significant potential risks to the patient's health. If surgery is required it should generally be less than 2.0. For simple surgical procedures, INR less than 2.5 is generally safe. If INR is higher than the level desired, the physician may elect to change anticoagulant therapy. Often, it is discontinued for 2–3 days before the treatment and INR is checked on the day of therapy. If found to be in the acceptable range, the dentist may proceed with the treatment and the anticoagulant is resumed immediately after treatment.

Patients with congenital bleeding disorders should be treated in specialist centers where cooperation between surgeon and hematologist is established.

Epilepsy

Epilepsy is a term that describes a group of disorders characterized by chronic, recurrent, paroxysmal changes in neurologic function that are caused by abnormal electrical activity in the brain. The most significant oral complication is gingival overgrowth associated with phenytoin. The anterior labial surfaces of the maxillary and mandibular gingiva are most commonly and severely affected.

The first step in the management is recording a proper medical history regarding the seizures, the type, age of onset, cause and medications currently being used. The appointments should be scheduled in the morning and before initiating the process make sure that the patient has taken his medication. Epileptics can have good and bad phases and dental treatment should be carried out in a good phase, when attacks are infrequent. A consultation with the physician is advised before dental treatment in poorly controlled patients. They may require additional anticonvulsant or sedative medications. Mouth prop is to be used during dental treatment. Keep equipment as much as possible away from the area of the patient. Be alert for any feature that may indicate the start of seizure. Aspirin and NSAIDs should not be administered to patients taking valproic acid. Propoxyphene and erythromycin should not be administered to patients taking carbamazepine.

Bronchial Asthma

Bronchial asthma is a generalized airway obstruction due to bronchial muscle contraction, mucosa swelling and increased mucus production, which in the early stages is paroxysmal and reversible. Exposure to allergens and/or stress can induce an attack. Infrequent attacks of asthma can be managed by salbutamol inhalers or can be used prophylactically, if an attack is predicted. e.g. before exercise or prior to a stressful event such as dental treatment. If the attacks are more frequent, then salbutamol should be used regularly. If this is insufficient, inhaled steroids (or cromoglycate in the young) should be used. In severe cases systemic steroids may be prescribed. Patients on steroid inhalers are prone to oral and pharyngeal thrush and those on ipratropium bromide may complain of dry mouth.

During dental treatment, avoid anxiety which may precipitate an asthmatic attack and advise the patients to bring their regular medication with them. Elective dental care should be deferred in severe asthmatics until they are in a better phase. Patient should not be treated during sickness, e.g. flu-like symptoms. These patients may present with frequent allergy to penicillin. Epinephrine, erythromycin, clindamycin and azithromycin are contraindicated for patients on theophylline. Aspirin and NSAIDs should be avoided as they precipitate the asthmatic attack. LA containing vasoconstrictor should be avoided, as some patients may react to sulphites present as preservatives in it. Avoid antihistamines such as promethazine and diphenhydramine as they cause a drying effect which can exacerbate the formation of tenacious mucus in acute attack.

Renal Diseases

Renal disease in children mainly comprises the so-called nephritic syndromes which may progress to chronic renal failure (CRF). Progression to CRF leads to the need for dialysis and possibly transplantation. CRF patients may be taking corticosteroid and other immunosuppression drugs. This can make medical management difficult for these patients. Retarded teeth eruption can be demonstrated in children with renal failure.

Potential problems in these patients include anemia, bleeding tendencies, associated anticoagulant therapy, impaired drug excretion, hypertension, infections such as hepatitis B and renal osteodystrophy. The main are of concern is the bleeding tendency. Careful hemostasis should be ensured, if surgery is necessary. The greatest foe in these patients is infection. Hence, teeth with severe bone loss, furcation, attachment loss, abscesses or requiring extensive surgical procedures should be extracted, leaving a maintainable oral cavity. Local anesthesia is safe unless there is severe bleeding tendency. Prophylactic antibiotics are to be prescribed due to immunosuppression. Tetracycline should be avoided in chronic renal failure. Aspirin and NSAIDs should be avoided as they affect renal function. Codeine and dihydrocodeine are favored as analgesics and diazepam may be used. Dry mouth and decreased salivary flow result in calculus accumulation. Alter the dosage of drugs eliminated by kidney such as penicillin.

The patients undergoing dialysis requires modifications in the treatment plan. There are 3 modes of dialysis namely, intermittent peritoneal dialysis, chronic ambulatory dialysis and hemodialysis, of which only hemodialysis patients require special precautions. They are at a higher risk for viral hepatitis, anemia and prolonged hemorrhage. Such patients should be screened for hepatitis B and C before any therapy. Antibiotic prophylaxis should be provided to prevent endarteritis of the AV shunt or fistula. Dental treatment is best carried out on the day after dialysis, when the effects of heparinization have subsided. If any uremic problems such as uremic stomatitis develop, the patient should be referred to a physician. If oral infections do not resolve promptly, then refer to the physician to prevent systemic dissemination.

Liver Disorders

Liver disorders are important to the dentist due to a potential bleeding tendency, intolerance to drugs (e.g. general anesthetics, benzodiazepines) and the possibility of underlying infective causes for the liver dysfunction. They may range from mild conditions to complete liver failure. Signs of liver disease include jaundice, spider nevi, leukonychia, finger-clubbing, palmar erythema, Dupuytren's contracture, among others. Patients with parenchymal liver disease have impaired hemostasis and can present serious bleeding problems as liver is the site of production for most of the clotting factors.

Disorders associated with an early rise in serum levels of conjugated bilirubin can cause dental hypoplasia and greenish discoloration of the teeth. LA is safe given in normal doses, but prilocaine or articaine are preferred to lidocaine. Severe bleeding can occur after dental extractions in patients with chronic liver disease and hence the clotting status must be tested. The most common liver function test (LFT) involves the measurement of aspartate transaminase (AST) and alanine transaminase (ALT). ALT may also be raised in cardiac or skeletal muscle damage and is therefore not specific for liver disease.

The use of any drug in a patient with severe liver disease should be discussed with the patient's physician. Many drugs are metabolized in the liver; hence hepatic impairment will lead to failure of metabolism of these drugs that can result in toxicity. In some cases, dose reduction is required, while in others drugs should be avoided completely. Erythromycin, metronidazole and tetracyclines should be avoided. The anti-fungal drug miconazole is contraindicated, if there is hepatic impairment and fluconazole requires dose reduction. Antimicrobials such as penicillin, cephalexin and cefazolin can be safely given in normal doses. Acetaminophen can be used for analgesia in lower than normal doses. Aspirin and NSAIDs should be avoided because of the risk of gastric hemorrhage.

Hepatitis B

Since majority of hepatitis infections are undiagnosed, the clinician must be aware of high-risk groups, such as renal dialysis patients, immunosuppressed patients, patients receiving multiple blood transfusions, healthcare workers, homosexuals, drug addicts and hospitalized patients. The main concerns in these patients are highly infective disease, bleeding tendency and drug sensitivity. Pure saliva does not contain HBsAg, but serum via gingival exudates does. Blood, plasma or serum can be infectious as little as 0.0000001 mL of HBsAg. The only oral complication associated with hepatitis is the potential for abnormal bleeding in cases of significant liver damage. If surgery is required, it is advisable to:

- Check the PT. If it is >35 minutes, an injection of vitamin K will usually correct the problem. This should be discussed with the patient's physician.
- Monitor the bleeding time to check platelet function. If it is not <20 minutes, the patient may require platelet replacement before surgery. This should also be discussed with the patient's physician.

Dentist should treat the patient within the current regulations for cross infection control. Patients with active acute hepatitis B should have dental treatment after complete recovery only, which takes about 3 months after symptomatic recovery, unless the situation is an emergency. In an emergency case, consult the patient's physician regarding status. Since hepatitis may alter coagulation, measure PT and BT, if bleeding is likely to occur during or after treatment. Change the treatment accordingly. All personnels should use full barrier technique, including masks, gloves, eye shields and disposable gowns. Use disposable covers for light and drawer handles, trays and also cover the headrest. All disposable items and covers should be bagged after treatment, labeled and disposed following proper guidelines for disposal of biohazardous waste. Needle stick injury can transmit the virus. An injection of hepatitis B immunoglobulin (HBIG) within 24 hours of contact may protect from developing hepatitis. Aerosol production should be minimized by not using ultrasonic instruments, air syringe or high speed handpieces as saliva contains a distillate of the virus. It is highly recommended to pre-rinse for 30 seconds with chlorhexidine gluconate.

If a patient is found to be a hepatitis B carrier, recommendations from the Center for Disease Control (CDC) for avoiding transmission of infection should be closely followed. In addition, some hepatitis carriers may have chronic active hepatitis, leading to compromised liver function and interfering with hemostasis and drug metabolism. Physician consultation or laboratory screening for liver function is advised. Any patient having signs or symptoms suggesting hepatitis should be referred to a physician, and should not be treated. If emergency care becomes necessary, it should be provided similar to the patient with acute disease.

Patients Receiving Steroid Therapy

General dental procedures for patients receiving long-term steroid medication do not warrant supplementation with additional glucocorticoids. Patients undergoing minor surgical procedures under local anesthesia are at very low risk for developing adrenal crisis and such patients should maintain their usual dose of glucocorticoids. However, those patients taking high doses of steroid should double the usual dose on the day.

Unexplained hypotension in patients on exogenous steroids should be investigated for other possible causes, because adrenal crisis is rare and patients on glucocorticoids are at high risk of various other medical complications. If adrenal insufficiency is suspected, secondary adrenal disease needs to be ruled out. Glucocorticoid therapy will cause adrenal suppression that affects adrenal functions for up to 12 months, but the patients stress response will return within 14–30 days. Accordingly, a number of guidelines for managing dental patients who either have been or are presently taking corticosteroids are suggested:

General Guidelines

Dental Treatment with Local Anesthetics

- *Patients who have taken glucocorticoids in the past but are presently not taking any type of glucocorticoid therapy:* Although adrenal suppression would be present, no study has shown nonfunctional stress response days after cessation of therapy. Therefore, there is no need for replacement therapy for dental treatment in patients who have not taken glucocorticoids during the preceding 30 days. If treatment is necessary during the first 30 days, treat the patient as if he were completely adrenally suppressed and without a normal stress response.

- *Patients who have been receiving alternate day therapy for at least 30 days:* During the offdays the patient will display abnormal response to stress stimuli. If possible, treat patient receiving alternate day therapy on an off day. In such cases, no replacement therapy will be necessary.
- *Patients receiving daily glucocorticoid therapy:* Patients receiving daily low dose corticosteroid therapy (below 30 mg hydrocortisone equivalent) will not need replacement therapy.

Dental Procedures with General Anesthesia

- *Patients who are presently not receiving any type of glucocorticoid therapy but who have taken glucocorticoids in the past:* 30 days after cessation of therapy, no replacement therapy is needed. If treatment is necessary with in the first 30 days after cessation of therapy, a steroid preparation (50 mg hydrocortisone administered IM at midnight, 100 mg hydrocortisone given IM when the patient is called to the operating room in the morning and 10 mg hydrocortisone/hr during the operation) should be used. Titrate down with dosage during the recovery period according to the post-operative pain induced stress levels.
- *Patients who have been receiving alternate day therapy for at least 30 days:* Schedule the operation on an off-day. There is no need for replacement therapy, but follow-up for signs of recurrence of the underlying disease. If it is necessary to perform the operation during an on day, a steroid preparation and titration of the dose down to the regular dosage is advisable.
- *Patients receiving daily glucocorticoid therapy:* Consult the patient's physician and always use a steroid preparation. Titrate the patient down to the normal dosage. The main complication of this therapy is the risk of precipitating an acute adrenal crisis in situations of stress. Therefore, patient must always be administered preoperative steroid cover to ensure circulating levels of corticosteroids are sufficient to meet the needs of the body.

As a general rule, adrenocortical function is likely to be suppressed, if:

- The patient is currently taking corticosteroids in excess of 7.5 mg prednisolone (or equivalent dose of any corticosteroid) daily.
- Corticosteroids have been taken regularly for more than a month in the last year.
- There has been extensive use of topical corticosteroids by the patient.

However, all patients should be considered individually taking into consideration the disease process for which the medication is prescribed, duration and dosage of corticosteroid therapy and procedure to be undertaken.

For patients at risk of a steroid crisis, the administration of supplemental steroid, in the form of hydrocortisone, is undertaken to mimic the stress response. Under major stress, circulating cortisol levels will not exceed 300 mg in 24 hours (the normal level is approximately 20 mg/24 hours). Therefore, the actual dose used for the prophylaxis of adrenal crisis is estimated **(Table 4)**.

Table 4: Estimation of steroid cover for different conditions

	No steroids for previous 12 months	*Steroids taken during previous 12 months*	*Steroids currently being taken*
Conservative dentistry	No cover required	Give hydrocortisone 200 mg orally or IV preoperatively.	Give hydrocortisone 200 mg orally or IV preoperatively. Continue normal steroid medication after surgery.
Intermediate surgery (multiple extraction or surgery under general anesthesia).	Consider coverage, if large doses of steroid were given. Test adrenocortical function (ACTH stimulation test).	Give hydrocortisone 200 mg IV preoperatively and IM 6 hourly for 24 hours.	Give hydrocortisone 200 mg IV preoperatively and IM 6 hourly for 24 hours, then continue normal medication.

Dental Management Guidelines for Patients with Adrenal Insufficiency

- Schedule elective procedures surgery in the morning, when cortisol levels usually are highest.
- Define the risk of adrenal insufficiency through medical history and clinical examination. An increased risk of adrenal insufficiency exists when there is a history of tuberculosis or HIV infection, since opportunistic infectious agent can attack the adrenal glands.
- Ensure that patients with adrenal insufficiency take their usual glucocorticoid dose before a stressful surgical procedure. Provide proper stress reduction, since anxiety can increase cortisol demand.
- Avoid general anesthesia for outpatient procedures, since it increases glucocorticoid demand. Avoid the use of barbiturates, since these drugs increase the metabolism of cortisol and reduce blood levels of cortisol.
- Use of nitrous oxide oxygen or IV or oral benzodiazepine sedation is helpful, since plasma cortisol levels are not reduced by these agents.
- Minor surgeries require minimal steroid coverage. The patient's usual daily dose typically is sufficient.
- Major surgeries and those lasting more than a hour or involving general anesthesia should be performed in a hospital with steroid supplementation.
- Discontinue drug therapy that decreases cortisol levels (e.g. ketoconazole) at least 24 hours before surgery, with the physician's consent.
- Provide adequate pain control during the operative and postoperative phase of care by administering long acting local anesthetics (e.g. bupivacaine) at the end of the procedure, as well as regular analgesic dosing.
- Use mild sedatives for apprehensive patients.
- Blood and other fluid volume loss, as well as the use of anticoagulants can exacerbate hypotension and increase the risk of adrenal insufficiency like symptoms. Thus, methods to reduce blood loss should be used.

- Monitor blood pressure throughout the procedure and before the patient leaves the dental office. Patients whose pressure is at or below 100/60 mm Hg should receive fluid replacement (5% dextrose), vasopressors or if needed glucocorticoids.
- Elective dental surgery procedures should be postponed until steroid therapy is discontinued or modifications are explored with the prescribing physician. If the dental procedure, such as emergency tooth extraction, cannot be delayed it should be limited to localized regions in order to minimize the size of the wound. All possible safeguards should be employed to prevent contamination of the site and prophylactic antibiotics should be administered.
- Every patient undergoing dental therapy should be questioned whether he has been prescribed glucocorticoids in the past or is administered presently.
- If it is determined that the patient is currently taking a systemic glucocorticoid medication, additional information regarding dosage, route of administration, frequency of doses and duration of therapy is necessary. If a patient is not presently taking glucocorticoids but has in the past, the length of time since the medication was last received is equally crucial.
- Patients receiving glucocorticoid in doses greater than the equivalent of 30 mg of cortisone daily for a continuous period of 1 week or longer have a possibility of developing adrenal crisis. The higher the daily dosage, the longer the period of administration or the shorter the period since discontinuation the greater the potential risk of adrenal crisis. Persons who have discontinued this type of therapy with in the past year are also at risk.
- If it is decided that dental procedures must be performed, consultation with the prescribing physician is mandatory. If the patient has a risk of adrenal crisis, 2 precautions should be undertaken: (1) Increased administration of glucocorticoids and (2) Stress reduction.
- This can be achieved by administration of steroid prep. A steroid prep is a controlled increase of glucocorticoids given prior to the patients' dental appointment which is slowly reduced to a normal dosage level over a 2–3 day period following therapy.
- Dentist must carefully evaluate the extent of dental procedures and estimate the apprehension of patients prior to discussing their recommendations with physicians.

The guideline that may be used to categorize management in such patients has been mentioned in **Table 5**.

Prosthetic Joint Replacement

The main treatment consideration for such patients relates to the potential need for antibiotic prophylaxis before any dental treatment. However, very few cases have been reported to cause prosthetic joint infections due to dental-induced bacteremia. Hence, the American Dental Association, American Academy of Orthopedic Surgeons, American Academy of Oral Medicine and British Society for Antimicrobial Chemotherapy, all agree that a routine antibiotic

Table 5: Guidelines used to categorize management

Category I	
Routine noninvasive dental therapy (examination, impressions, etc.), a non-apprehensive patient and slight risk of pituitary adrenal suppression.	• No steroid preparation is required
Category II	
Routine invasive dental therapy (restoration, routine endodontics, scaling and root planning, biopsy) or a moderately apprehensive patient or relatively greater risk of pituitary adrenal suppression	• A steroid prep consisting of doubling the daily dosage of glucocorticoid prior to the procedure followed by gradually reducing the dose each day for 3 days back to the normal dosage. • Light to moderate sedation.
Category III	
Combination of two or more factors from category II or extensive invasive dental therapy (long restorative or endodontic procedures, multiple extractions, periodontal or endodontic surgery) or an extremely apprehensive patient or severe risk of pituitary adrenal suppression.	• A steroid prep consisting of quadrupling the daily dosage of glucocorticoids prior to the procedure followed by gradual reduction over a 2 or 3 day period to the normal dosage.
Category IV	
Combination of two or more of the situations in category III or a long-surgical procedure.	• Hospitalization of the patient where administration of extensive doses of glucocorticoids, heavy sedation and appropriate monitoring can be provided. • All administration of steroid prep should be by mutual agreement with the physician in charge of glucocorticoids therapy. • Everyday 24–30 mg of cortisol (equivalent to 5–7.5 mg prednisolone) is released in a rhythmic pulsatile approach. Under stress, this may increase to 300 mg (60 mg prednisolone equivalent) per day.

prophylaxis before dental treatment is not indicated in most patients with such joint replacements. However, prophylaxis is indicated in all patients within the first 2 years after the replacement and for high-risk patients, that includes those with previous prosthetic joint infections, rheumatoid arthritis, SLE, immunosuppression, type I diabetes, hemophilia and malnourishment. Consult the patient's orthopedic surgeon before the treatment to assess the risk for joint infection relative to current dental status and type of treatment planned. The suggested antibiotic regimens for prevention of prosthetic joint infections are given in **Table 6**.

Table 6: Suggested antibiotic regimens for prevention of prosthetic joint infections

Situation	*Drugs*
Patients not allergic to penicillin	Cephalexin, cepharidine or amoxicillin 2 g orally 1 hour prior to the treatment
Patients allergic to penicillin	Clindamycin 600 mg orally 1 hour prior to the treatment
Patients not allergic to penicillin, but unable to take oral medication	Cefazolin 1 g or ampicillin 2 g IM or IV 1 hour prior to the treatment
Patients allergic to penicillin, and unable to take oral medication	Clindamycin 600 mg IV 1 hour prior to the treatment (must be diluted and injected slowly)

HIV and AIDS

Similar to hepatitis, not all HIV-infected patients know that they are infected when they report for dental treatment and some known patients may not admit their status during medical history. Therefore, every patient who receives dental treatment should be managed as a potentially infected person, using universal precautions for all therapy. Extensive treatment plans must be considered keeping in mind the patient's systemic health, prognosis and survival time. Selection of an appropriate treatment plan depends on the state of the overall health of the patient, as there occurs large variations in the progression of the disease. An awareness of oral disorders associated with HIV infection may allow the clinician to recognize previously undiagnosed cases or to modify treatment plan accordingly.

Tuberculosis

These patients should receive only emergency care, following the guidelines as mentioned for hepatitis. If the patient has completed chemotherapy, it is essential to medical clearance regarding infectivity and the results of sputum cultures for *Mycobacterium tuberculosis*. Once the cultures are negative and medical clearance is obtained, normal treatment protocol may be followed. Adequate treatment of tuberculosis requires 18 months, followed by thorough post-treatment follow-up that includes chest radiographs, sputum cultures and a review of patient's symptoms by the physician every 12 months at least. Any patient with irregular medical follow-up and suspected signs and symptoms should be referred for evaluation.

9

Management of Medical Emergencies

Introduction

Medical emergencies can occur at any time in the dental office. They can happen to anyone, from the anxious patient in the reception room to the elderly diabetic who was asked to skip breakfast prior to coming for the appointment. They can happen to the receptionist with an epileptic disorder or to the dentist experiencing prolonged chest discomfort. It is estimated that the average dentist will have to deal with one or two life-threatening medical emergencies during their career. Knowing how to handle medical emergencies will make the dental practitioners more confident in his or her ability to handle all aspects of the job.

The best way to handle an emergency is to be prepared in advance. All healthcare providers should be prepared to recognize and handle medical emergencies in the office. Staff should be trained and frequently updated in first aid and cardiopulmonary resuscitation procedures. A written emergency plan should be available, and all staff members should be thoroughly familiar with it and their responsibilities in an emergency. This includes training of dental hygienists, auxillaries and other aids in handling emergencies, development and posting of emergency guidelines, and maintenance of an emergency kit, fully equipped and ready for immediate use.

Most emergencies can be prevented by adequate preparation of the patient and staff. The following are the suggested guidelines:

- A medical history of every patient should be obtained and updated at subsequent visits. The patients' physician consultation should be obtained where required.
- Ask the patients to take their normal medications on the day of their appointment and schedule the appointments accordingly. Cardiac and asthmatic patients should carry their inhalers or nitroglycerin tablets in the event an asthma or angina attack is precipitated by the stress of dental treatment. Appointments for diabetic patients should be scheduled around meal time.
- Assistants and staff members should be well trained to monitor and interpret vital signs. These should be taken at the initial visit and at each subsequent visit for patients may be at risk.
- All staff members should be trained in basic first aid procedures and basic life support (CPR).

- There should be a written emergency plan in the clinics and dental offices and each staff member should know and practice their particular function in an emergency. Emergency telephone numbers should be kept handy.
- Office personnel should be aware of the signs and symptoms indicating an emergency. Each office should have an emergency kit readily available.
- All staff should be aware of their legal responsibilities when responding to an office emergency.

Remember, the best handled medical emergency will always be the one that never happened.

Patient History

Prevention and preparation are often the best antidotes for an emergency. The increasing numbers of older patients with significant medical problems requiring dental treatment, longer appointments, and the increasing use of new medications with complex interactions all increase the risk of a life-threatening problem occurring during the treatment. The majority of medical emergencies, however, can be anticipated and avoided with appropriate risk reduction by recording a proper medical and family history and recording of vital signs to identify the risk patients.

The medical history should include information regarding the patient's past and present health status. It should also include questions indicating problems the patient may not be aware of, but which may alter treatment. A number of medical problems may alter dental treatment. Additional information on questions answered in the affirmative to a health issue should be obtained. A list of medication names and dosages that are currently prescribed to the patient and drug allergies, if any should also be recorded. Additional questions should be asked regarding the use of any herbal medicines. To keep the health history current, the patient should be questioned about any changes in their general health since their last visit. A list of medical conditions and drugs that may affect the dental treatment has been given in **Tables 1 and 2**.

Vital Signs

Obtaining vital signs is not frequently seen in dental offices. This provides a baseline measurement from which alterations in the patient's condition can be determined. These include measurement of blood pressure, pulse, respirations, and temperature prior to each treatment. The recording of vital signs has been discussed earlier in Chapter 5.

Office Emergency Plan

Because it is impossible to know when an emergency may occur or what form it may take, it is important that every dental office have an established, written, and practiced routine for handling emergencies. Emergency numbers such as 102 should be posted conspicuously at every phone in the set-up. Other phone numbers for emergencies might include the hospital emergency department, an oral surgeon, a physician, and so forth.

Table 1: Few medical conditions that may alter dental treatment

Syncope	Stress may provoke fainting spells, an ammonia inhalant should always be available at chair side
Asthma/chronic obstructive pulmonary disease	Patient should keep the inhaler available during treatment, and sometimes may need puff before treatment. Nitrous oxide sedation should be used with caution
Difficulty during breathing	Patient may have present with difficulty on lying supine in the dental chair
Cardiac ailments	Noted chest pain, angina, or heart problem history should put the dental practitioner on alert. Sublingual nitroglycerin tablets must be available. Certain heart problems require antibiotic prophylaxis before any dental treatment can be initiated.
Hypertension	Anesthetics with epinephrine could elevate blood pressure
Hypotension	Orthostatic hypotension may develop when moving patient from supine to sitting or standing position
Hyperventilation	Advising the patient to breathe into a paper bag is no longer the preferred treatment. The patient should be talked through it and calmed while counting the number of breaths.
Diabetes	Instant glucose should be available for hypoglycemic reactions.
Glaucoma	Atropine used as an anti-sialagogue could increase pressure in the anterior chamber of the eye. Caution must be used when prescribing medicines that could increase eye pressure.
Adrenal insufficiency	If the patient is lacking cortisol, or is on extensive steroid therapy, stress may lead to a crisis
Hemophilia	Consult the patient's physician before treatment which may result in bleeding.
Jaundice	May cause complications such as hepatitis, liver disease, and alcoholic cirrhosis.
Epilepsy	Often associated triggers to induce a seizure. Phenytoin prescribed patients will present with gingival hyperplasia.
Allergies	Patients with any allergic conditions are more prone to drug allergies
Pregnancy	The patient should be protected from radiation, cannot be laid supine in the third trimester, as there may be a risk to develop supine hypotension. Drugs and anesthetics should be prescribed with caution due to placental transfer.
Psychiatric illness	Patients may be prone to syncope, anxiety, bizarre reactions to common events. Nitrous oxide sedation may cause problems in such patients.
Sinus Problems	Drainage and breathing difficulties can develop during treatment
Chemotherapy/ radiation therapy/ organ transplants	Consult the treating physicians before initiating the dental procedure, as the patients may be prone to infection or bone disorders
Tuberculosis	Treatment should only be completed in a hospital setting and only for emergency procedures

Table 2: Drugs which may alter dental treatment	
Acetylsalicylic acid (Aspirin) and warfarin (Coumadine)	These act as blood thinner and increase the risk of bleeding.
Antibiotics (Penicillins, cephalosporins, macrolides, sulfonamides)	These are prescribed for preventive measures and to treat oral infection, but can cause xerostomia.
Phenytoin (Dilantin)	Prescribed to treat seizures, gingival hyperplasia
Nitroglycerin (Nitrostate, Nitro-Bide)	Chest pain, angina and heart attack
Insulin	Identifies Type I diabetes patients who are prone to hypoglycemia
Digitalis (Digoxine, Lanoxine)	Treats abnormal heart rate and arrhythmias, irregular pulse, ankle swelling and fluid retention indicating heart failure

A code word or phrase indicating an emergency should be determined. This will alert other staff to the existence of an emergency and avoid possible upset to patients in nearby operatories or in the reception area. Every member of the dental staff should have a specific assignment in an emergency. The number of assignments and specific functions will be determined by staff size and training. The office emergency plan should be updated and practiced regularly at periodic meetings or following annual CPR training sessions. Mock scenarios of various emergency situations can be developed which will allow each staff member to act out their assigned roles.

With careful planning and frequent practice of the office emergency plan, confusion and panic can be significantly reduced during an actual emergency.

Emergency Training

Every member of the dental team should have completed a basic first aid course and have annual training in cardiopulmonary resuscitation. The CPR course for healthcare providers is recommended because it includes two-person CPR, child and infant CPR, and the use of a mask. Studies have shown that if CPR skills are not used regularly, they are soon forgotten and hence the practitioners and staff should be annually trained for the skills. Masks with one-way valves should be used in training and supplied to office personnel for actual patient use as specified by OSHA regulations. Bag-valve-mask devices are more difficult for the occasional user to actually ventilate a patient with such a device. Pocket masks are much easier to use, provide effective ventilations, and have ports for the addition of supplemental oxygen. A basic first aid course provides the staff with information on emergency care in common injury situations. Topics such as the control of bleeding, treatment of burns, and the handling of sprains and fractures are covered in such courses.

Cardiopulmonary Resuscitation

The 2010 AHA Guidelines for Cardiopulmonary Resuscitation (CPR) recommend a change in the Basic Life Support (BLS) sequence of steps from A-B-C (Airway, Breathing, Chest compressions) to C-A-B (Chest compressions, Airway, Breathing) for adults, children, and infants (excludes newborns). This fundamental change in the CPR sequence will require re-education of everyone who has ever learned CPR, but the benefit will justify the effort.

Here is a step-by-step guide for the new CPR:
- Call emergency or 102.
- Try to get the person to respond; if he does not, roll the person on his or her back.
- Start chest compressions. Place the heel of your hand on the center of the victim's chest. Put your other hand on top of the first with your fingers interlaced.
- Press down so you compress the chest at least 2 inches in adults and children, and 1.5 inches in infants. "One hundred times a minute or even a little faster is optimal," Sayre says.
- If you have been trained in CPR, you can now open the airway with a head tilt and chin lift.
- Pinch closed the nose of the victim. Take a normal breath, cover the victim's mouth with yours to create an airtight seal, and then give two, one-second breaths as you watch for the chest to rise.
- Continue compressions and breaths—30 compressions, 2 breaths—until help arrives.

An automatic external defibrillator (AED) is an adjunct piece of equipment every dental clinic should consider having available as part of the office emergency kit. The AED is a computerized defibrillator that recognizes the presence of ventricular fibrillation or rapid ventricular tachycardia and then allows the operator to administer "shocks" to convert the patient's heart rhythm back to normal. For every minute that lapses before defibrillation, the survival rate decreases by 10%. The AED is equipped with a voice prompt to lead the operator through its usage and requires no special training.

Initial Emergency Procedures

Physical signs and symptoms that may indicate an incipient medical emergency include chest pain, pale skin, sweating, vomiting, irregular respiratory rate, altered or unusual sensations, hemorrhage, and changes in pulse and blood pressure.

When an emergency situation is recognized, dental treatment should be stopped immediately and assistance summoned. If the patient was receiving nitrous oxide, it should be discontinued. 100% oxygen should be given in its place in every case but hyperventilation. Establish patient responsiveness by shaking and asking in a loud voice "Are you okay?" Lay the patient in a supine position. If the situation appears serious, call emergency immediately.

Check for the presence of a carotid pulse for 5–10 seconds. If no pulse is present, lay the patient flat in the chair with a board behind the chest. If this is not possible move the patient to the floor and begin chest compressions on a bared chest. Leaving the patient in the chair with a board behind the chest lessens the chance of injury that may happen by moving the patient to the floor. If the pulse is present, check the rate and strength. Begin fast chest compressions according to the new CPR guidelines. Apply the defibrillator pads of the AED as soon as it arrives, turn the unit "on" and follow the voice prompt directions. In a pulseless patient, defibrillation takes precedence over chest compressions.

Open the patient's airway using the head-tilt chin-lift, remove any dental materials from the patient's mouth, and suction as necessary. Assess for spontaneous breathing for 3 to 5 seconds. If the patient is not breathing, give 2 slow breaths via a pocket mask.

The initial emergency steps are summarized as follows:

- *Recognition:*
  - Stop dental treatment
  - Call for help and emergency kit
  - Assess consciousness; if unconscious, recline chair with legs above head
  - Discontinue nitrous oxide, administer 100% oxygen in all cases but hyperventilation
- *Assess circulation*:
  - Check for pulse
  - If NO pulse, lay the patient flat with board beneath chest or move patient to floor and begin chest compressions
  - Apply the AED
  - If pulse is present, check rate and strength
- *Airway*:
  - Open airway
  - Use head tilt-chin lift
  - Suction as necessary
- *Breathing*:
  - Check for breathing
  - If no breathing, give 2 breaths via pocket mask (100% O_2, if possible)
  - Insert oral airway, if apnea
  - Call for the AED
- *Assess patient and situation*:
  - Manage situation as appropriate to diagnosis
  - Take and record vital signs for breathing with pulse
  - Never attempt to transport the patient yourself
  - *Call emergency immediately for any of the following*: Cardiac arrest, if chest pain persists for more than 5 minutes and is not relieved by nitroglycerin, respiratory arrest, unconsciousness for greater than a minute, prolonged confusion state, respiratory difficulty, seizures, systolic blood pressure < 100 mm Hg or pulse > 120 beats/minute.
  - Use judgment for conditions not mentioned earlier

- Treat patient supportively until emergency help arrives
- Have medical history and patient medications available for rescue squad. Inform rescue squad of recorded vital signs, initiated treatments and any medications given.

Anxiety Reduction

Stress is the major factor causing medical emergencies in the dental office. Syncope, hyperventilation, seizures, asthma attacks, and angina are some of the more common emergencies and they all can be precipitated by stress and anxiety. These problems are fairly easy to prevent. The first step is to identify the patient likely to experience anxiety. Anxious patients tend to startle easily, have a rapid heart rate, exhibit pale and clammy skin, and appear apprehensive. In pre-treatment conversations, they may relate worry about the appointment or indicate a fear of pain.

Once identified, steps can be taken to manage the anxiety proactively. A first step is to minimize the amount of waiting prior to any procedure. The procedure should be explained to the patient in a thorough and detailed manner, so that he or she experiences no surprise in the operatory. In more extreme cases, patients may need to be premedicated with anti-anxiety agents. Adequate pain control should be used and longer procedures should be divided into shorter dental appointments.

Aspiration and Choking

The patients present with the following signs and symptoms:

- Patient may cough and splutter
- May complain of breathing difficulty and breathing may become noisy on inspiration
- Patient may develop paradoxical chest or abdominal movements
- Patient may become cyanosed and lose consciousness

Management

In cases of aspiration encourage the patient to cough vigorously. Administer 100% oxygen, flow rate: 10 liter/minute. Administer a salbutamol inhaler, 4 puffs (100 μg/actuation), through a large-volume spacer, repeat as needed.

If you suspect that a large fragment has been inhaled or swallowed but there are no signs or symptoms, refer the patient to hospital for X-ray and removal of the fragment, if necessary. If the patient is symptomatic following aspiration, refer to the hospital as an emergency.

In cases of choking remove any visible foreign bodies in the mouth and pharynx, and encourage the patient to cough. If the patient is unable to cough but remains conscious, commence back blows followed by abdominal thrusts. If the patient becomes unconscious, basic life support should be started immediately this may also help to dislodge the foreign body. Call an ambulance and transfer patient to hospital as an emergency.

Anaphylaxis

An allergic reaction is the result of an antigen-antibody reaction to a substance to which the patient has been previously sensitized. Histamine and other complex chemicals are released from body cells causing symptoms in the patient. These symptoms may be confined to a single organ system or become generalized as in the case of anaphylaxis. The most likely allergens in the dental set-up are exposures to latex, local anesthetics, or antibiotics, however, certain food products to which the patient had prior to the appointment such as nuts, shellfish, milk products, and strawberries may trigger the allergic reaction.

Key Signs and Symptoms

- Angioneurotic edema (pharynx and upper airway), swelling of neck, hoarseness, stridor asthma (respiratory tract)
- Tachycardia (heart rate > 110 beats/minute)
- Urticaria—pruritus (integumentary system), itching, red skin
- Abdominal pain, vomiting, diarrhea, and a sense of impending doom
- Flushing, but pallor might also occur
- Patients may also display symptoms of mild allergy

Management

The priority is to transfer the patient to hospital as an emergency. Until help arrives assess the patient. Secure the patient's airway and help to restore their blood pressure by laying the patient flat and raising their feet. Administer 100% oxygen, flow rate: 10 liter/minute. Administer adrenaline, 0.5 mL (1:1000), intramuscular injection repeated after 5 minutes, if needed. The dosage of Adrenaline (1:1000) for children is as under:

- *6 months–6 years*: 0.15 mL
- *6–12 years*: 0.3 mL
- *12–18 years*: 0.5 mL
- Use 0.3 mL adrenaline for children aged 12–18 years, if the child is small or prepubertal.
- If cardiac arrest follows an anaphylactic reaction, start basic-life support immediately.

Mild Allergy

Key signs of mild allergy are as follows:

- Urticaria and rash, particularly of chest, hands and feet
- Rhinitis and conjunctivitis
- Mild bronchospasm without evidence of severe shortness of breath.

Management

Administer 1 Cetirizine tablet, 10 mg (Use with caution in patients with hepatic impairment or epilepsy). For children of 6-12 years, give Cetrizine tablet 10 mg or oral solution 5 mg/5 mL. Cetirizine tablets are not licensed for use in children less than 6 years, except for use in children aged 2–6 years for treatment of seasonal allergic rhinitis. For children of 12–18 years, dose is same as in adults.

Or

Administer 1 Chlorphenamine tablet, 4 mg. Chlorphenamine can cause drowsiness. Advise patients not to drive. Use with caution in patients with hepatic impairment, prostatic hypertrophy, epilepsy, urinary retention, glaucoma or pyloroduodenal obstruction. For children of 6–12 years give chlorphenamine tablet, 4 mg or oral solution 2 mg/5 mL. Avoid use in children with severe liver disease. Do not give to children under 2 years, except on specialist advice, because the safety of the use of chlorphenamine has not been established. For children of 12–18 years dose is same as in adults.

Or

Administer 1 Loratadine tablet 10 mg. Use with caution in patients with hepatic impairment or epilepsy. For children, give Loratadine tablet 10 mg and in children of 12–18 years, the dose is same as for adults.

If the patient displays signs of mild bronchospasm:

- Administer a salbutamol inhaler, 4 puffs (100 μg per actuation), through a large-volume spacer, repeat as needed.
- For children of 12–18 years administer salbutamol inhaler 1 puff via a spacer every 15 seconds (maximum 10 puffs), repeat above regimen at 10–20 minute intervals as needed.
- Refer the patient to their general medical practitioner.
- Treatment with antihistamines is only suitable in cases of mild allergy.

Asthma

Asthma is an allergic response of the bronchioles. It may affect any individual irrespective of age, but is more common in the younger age group. Patients may abruptly develop bronchospasm in response to anxiety and aerosolized particulate matter, which is evidenced by wheezing, coughing, and difficulty in breathing, and may also complain of chest tightness and develop cyanosis.

Signs of Life-threatening Asthma

- Cyanosis or respiratory rate <8 cycles/minute
- Bradycardia (heart rate <50 beats/minute)
- Exhaustion, confusion, decreased conscious level

Signs of Acute Severe Asthma

- Inability to complete sentences in one breath
- Respiratory rate >25 cycles/minute
- Tachycardia (heart rate >110 beats/minute)

Management

The priority is to transfer a patient displaying symptoms of life-threatening asthma to hospital immediately as an emergency. Assess the patient and make him sit in an upright position. Administer 100% oxygen, flow rate: 10 liter/

minute. Administer the patient's own bronchodilator (2 puffs); if unavailable, administer a salbutamol inhaler, 4 puffs (100 μg/actuation), through a large-volume spacer, repeat as needed. For children of 12–18 years administer salbutamol inhaler 1 puff via a spacer every 15 seconds (maximum 10 puffs), repeat above regimen at 10–20 minute intervals as needed.

If a patient suffering from a severe episode of asthma does not respond to treatment with bronchodilators within 5 minutes of administration, they should be transferred to hospital as an emergency.

Angina and Myocardial Infarction

The development of central chest discomfort frequently results from stressful situations in patients with coronary artery disease. In angina episodes, the coronary artery is unable to supply the heart muscle with adequate amounts of oxygenated blood, resulting in chest pain. The onset of anginal chest pain is usually directly related to exercise, stress, and anxiety. The decreased oxygen supply to the heart muscle is usually of short duration (less than 5 minutes) and no permanent damage occurs.

In myocardial infarction (MI or heart attack), a blood clot develops in one of the coronary arteries completely cutting-off blood supply to a portion of the heart muscle. Without a blood supply, the heart muscle dies within a few hours. The ischemic heart is very irritable and susceptible to cardiac arrhythmias. Whenever and wherever a myocardial infarction is recognized, emergency must be called immediately. This is critical, as about 50% of patients experiencing a MI will die in the first 2 hours.

Signs and Symptoms

- Progressive onset of severe, crushing pain in the centre and across the front of chest; the pain might radiate to the shoulders and down the arms (more commonly the left), into the neck and jaw or through to the back.
- Shortness of breath and increased respiratory rate
- Skin becomes pale and clammy
- Nausea and vomiting are common
- Pulse might be weak and blood pressure might fall

Management

Assess the patient and place the patient in whatever position is most comfortable. Administer 100% oxygen, flow rate: 10 liter/minute. Administer glyceryl trinitrate (GTN) spray, 2 puffs (400 μg per metered dose) sublingually, repeated after 3 minutes, if chest pain remains. If the patient has not previously had nitroglycerin, it is advisable to administer it while the patient is in a supine position, as hypotension is frequently seen in first time users. Calm and reassure the patient. If the patient does not respond to GTN treatment, then the priority is to transfer the patient to hospital as an emergency.

Initiate fibrinolysis, if possible, have patient chew 162 to 325 mg of dispersible aspirin. When chewed, the clinical effects are realized more quickly. If aspirin is given, send a note with the patient to inform the hospital staff. Aspirin is not licensed for use in children less than 16 years of age because, rarely, it can cause Reye's syndrome.

If the patient becomes unresponsive, check for signs of life (breathing and circulation), and if there are no signs of life or no normal breathing, initiate basic life support and carry out early defibrillation, if a defibrillator is available. The experience can be extremely frightening, with some patients voicing feelings of impending doom or death.

Cardiac Arrest

Of all the emergencies which may occur in the dental office cardiac arrest is certainly the most serious. It may result from an abnormal heart rhythm or secondary to a respiratory arrest. In either case, time and immediate intervention is of prime importance.

Signs

- Loss of consciousness
- Absence of breathing
- Loss of pulse
- Dilation of pupils

Management

The priority is to transfer the patient to hospital as an emergency. Call for an ambulance. Initiate basic life support, using 100% oxygen or ventilation, flow rate: 10 liter/minute. The rescuer should open the airway, look, listen, and feel for respirations. Next, check the carotid pulse for 5–10 seconds. If a pulse is absent, lay the patient flat with board beneath chest or move patient to floor. Begin the fast compressions for CPR as outlined earlier. Open the patient's airway using the head-tilt chin-lift. Remove any dental materials from the patient's mouth, and suction as necessary. Assess for spontaneous breathing for 3–5 seconds. If the patient is not breathing, give two slow breaths via a pocket mask. If a defibrillator is available, carry out early defibrillation.

Epilepsy

Convulsions or seizures are caused by waves of abnormal electrical activity in the brain in epileptic patients. As these waves spread across the surface of the brain, they stimulate other cells which are responsible for motor activity, sensation, or consciousness. These patients may have stopped taking or missed a dose of their anti-seizure medication or they may experience a seizure as a result of exposure to a triggered or stressful situation. It is important to note that otherwise normal patients may seize if the conditions are right, particularly with hypoglycemia or hypoxia.

Signs and Symptoms

- Sudden loss of consciousness, patient may become rigid, fall, might give a cry and becomes cyanosed (tonic phase)
- Jerking movements of the limbs; the tongue might be bitten (clonic phase)
- In some cases, the patient may have a premonition about having a seizure. This brief warning or aura may take the form of a strange smell, visual or auditory hallucination, or other strange sensation.
- Frothing from the mouth and urinary incontinence
- A seizure is followed by a period of drowsiness, confusion and extreme fatigue called the postictal phase.

Management

Assess the patient. Do not try to restrain convulsive movements. Ensure the patient is not at risk from injury. When observing a generalized motor seizure, never attempt to place or force any object between the patient's teeth. Bite sticks are ineffective and may cause damage to oral structures. Individuals experiencing a seizure exhibit incredible strength and attempts at restraint may result in fractures to the patient's bones. In addition, do not attempt to ventilate the patient during a seizure. Secure the patient's airway. Administer 100% oxygen, flow rate: 10 liters/minute

The seizure will typically last a few minutes; the patient might then become floppy but remain unconscious. Once the patient regains consciousness they may remain confused. However, if the epileptic fit is repeated or prolonged (5 minutes or longer), continue administering oxygen and administer 10 mg midazolam topically into the buccal cavity. Use either buccal liquid (10 mg/mL) or injection solution (5 mg/mL). For children of 10-18 years use the same dose as adults. For children of 6 months–1 year age administer 2.5 mg, for 1–5 years age group 5 mg and for 5–10 years administer 7.5 mg midazolam. Midazolam buccal liquid and midazolam injection solution are not licensed for use in status epilepticus

After convulsive movements have subsided, place the patient in the recovery position and check the airway. Do not send the patient home until they have recovered fully. Only give medication, if convulsive seizures are prolonged (last for 5 minutes or longer) or recur in quick succession. In these cases, and if this was the first episode of epilepsy for the patient, the convulsion was atypical, injury occurred or there is difficulty monitoring the patient, call for an ambulance.

Syncope

Fainting or syncope results from either the psychologic response to fear, anxiety, stress, pain, or unpleasant situations or from poor autonomic adjustments to changes in the patient's posture. In some cases, syncope may be due to very rapid or slow cardiac arrhythmias. Syncope accounts for over, 50% of reported emergencies in the dental set-up.

Signs and Symptoms

- Patient feels faint, dizzy, light-headed
- Slow pulse rate
- Loss of consciousness
- Pallor and sweating
- Nausea and vomiting

Management

Syncope can be prevented by identifying the patient prone to anxiety or who is using anti-anxiety agents. Fearful patients can be prescribed a premedication to help them relax for the appointment. Keep the patient supine if possible; with older patients, allow them time to slowly adjust to an upright posture after procedures are completed. In the elderly, rapid changes in posture can result in postural (orthostatic) hypotension.

When faced with a fainting episode, lay the patient flat and in supine position in the dental chair with the legs elevated. Loosen any tight clothing around the neck. Administer 100% oxygen, flow rate: 10 liters/minute until consciousness is regained. Do not allow the patient to sit up, as they will frequently faint again. Monitor vital signs. Because the patient regains consciousness almost immediately, the use of ammonia inhalants is unnecessary. It is recommended that treatment be stopped and rescheduled for another date.

Hypoglycemia

Hypoglycemia occurs when there is insufficient glucose in the bloodstream to meet the metabolic demands of cells. True hypoglycemia is seen only in Type I or in Type II diabetics using oral hypoglycemic agents. The lack of glucose in the neurons of the central nervous system results in immediate dysfunction. Hypoglycemia occurs when blood sugar levels drop below 80 mg/dL and typically becomes more acute in the 20–30 mg/dL range. If a source of glucose is not administered immediately, permanent damage may result.

Signs and Symptoms

- Patient appears confused and restless
- Patients may also complain of a headache or exhibit bizarre behavior
- Skin becomes pale, cool and clammy
- Heart rate increases
- On occasion, a patient may exhibit seizure activity or transient stroke-like symptoms.

Management

Hypoglycemia can be prevented by making sure the insulin dependent diabetic has eaten before treatment, by scheduling appointments in the morning, and by having a glucose source readily available at chair side. If the patient exhibits signs and symptoms of hypoglycemia, administer an oral carbohydrate such as regular cola, table sugar, or even a spoonful of honey or icing to raise blood glucose levels.

For a patient who becomes unconscious, maintain their airway, turn the patient on their side to prevent aspiration and administer glucose in the dependent cheek. This will usually provide sufficient glucose to allow the patient to regain consciousness. The patient should then drink a liquid high in sugar to increase their blood glucose level. Following a hypoglycemic reaction, advise the patient to eat a meal to maintain blood sugar levels and prevent a recurrence of the hypoglycemic episode.

Accidental Overdose

Rapid administration, excessive dosing, or inadvertent intravascular administration may all result in increased drug effects. Prevention is the key in avoiding adverse drug reactions. Ask the patient prior to the treatment about any allergies and hypersensitivity to any drugs.

If the drug is to be injected IV, administer it slowly, and use the minimum amount required to achieve the desired effect. When administering blocks, use an aspirating syringe. A child's bodysize and weight should be considered during dosing and anesthetic administration.

Most drugs have a few specific antidotes available. There are two notable exceptions. Narcan® (naloxone) is the antidote for accidental overdose of narcotics given IV such as Demerol® (meperidine). Narcan® can be used to reverse the hypotension, respiratory depression, and decreased level of consciousness caused by these narcotics. In the case of the benzodiazepines such as Valium® (diazepam) and Versed® (midazolam), a specific antidote-Romazicon® (flumazenil) is also available.

Management

The patient should be treated supportively until the effects of the drug wear off. Stop the administration of the drug, maintain the airway and ventilations monitor vital signs, and contact emergency, if the patient fails to show prompt improvement.

All of the toxic effects of lidocaine are due to its effects on the central nervous system and the conduction of nerve impulses. As there is no specific antidote for lidocaine toxicity, provide supportive care. Maintain the airway, administer oxygen, and treat other problems as they arise.

10

Checklist for Recording Patient's Data

Case History Porforma

Patient name: **OPD No:**

Age: **Sex:** **Date:**

Occupation: **Education:** **Martial status:**

Address:

Chief complaint:

History of present illness:

Dental history:

- Restoration
- Periodontal
- Endodontic
- Extractions or other surgical procedures
- Orthodontic
- Prosthodontic
- Other oral lesions

Complications, if any:

Medical history:

- Any serious illness:

  Cardiovascular
  Angina pectoris
  Myocardial infarction
  Congenital heart defect
  Rheumatic fever
  Hypertension
  Stroke
  CCF Edema of feet

  Respiratory
  Tuberculosis
  Asthma
  Shortness of breath
  Dyspnea
  Orthopnea
  Edema
  Other

  Endocrine
  Diabetes
  Thyroid disorders
  Parathyroid disorders
  Adrenal disorders
  Pituitary hormones
  Steroids
  Sex hormone therapy

  Hematopoietic
  Anemia
  Bleeding disorders
  Leukemia
  Other

  Gastrointestinal
  Ulcers
  Gastritis
  Bleeding
  Hyperacidity

  Liver
  Hepatitis
  Jaundice
  Cholecystitis
  Cirrhosis
  Other

Musculoskeletal
Bones
Muscles
Joints
TMJ

Neurologic
Epilepsy
Convulsions
Psychiatric
Paralysis
Shock
Faints/spells
Tranquilizers therapy

Genitourinary
Kidney disorders
Veneral diseases
Other

- Hospitalization, if any:
- Blood transfusion
  Quantity
  Cause
  Complications, if any:
- Allergies
  - Drugs
    Penicillin
    Sulfa drugs
    NSAIDs
    Cumarin derivatives
    Local anesthesia
    Barbiturates
    Analgesics: Opioids
  - Food stuff
  - Pollen grains
  - Dust
  - Others
- Menstrual/pregnancy/menopause:
- Medications
  Type and reason:
- Reviews of symptoms of systemic diseases of importance to the dentist
  - Diabetes mellitus
  - Liver diseases
  - Cardiovascular
  - Renal diseases
  - Neurologic/psychologic
  - Immunological

- Skin diseases
- Blood disorders
- ENT problems
- Infective disorders

- *Specialist opinion*:

Family history:

- Hemophilia
- Diabetes
- Hypertension
- Migraine
- Psychiatric
- Allergic diseases
- Neurologic
- Any other familial/inherited disorder
- History of any family member with similar problem?

Personal history:

Personal habits:	**Type**	**Frequency**	**Number**	**Duration**
– Smoking				
– Smokeless tobacco (with/without pan chewing)				
– Pan and betel nut chewing				
– Alcohol				

- **Habits related to oral hygiene**

– Method of brushing:	Toothbrush	Finger	Stick
– Material used:	Toothpaste Any other	Tooth powder	Charcoal
– Frequency of brushing:	Once	Twice	Thrice
– Time of brushing:	Before meals	After meals	
– Method of cleaning:	Vertical	Horizontal	Circular
– Frequency of changing the toothbrush:			
– Use of other oral Hygiene aids:	Floss	Interdental aids	Mouth wash

- **Habits related to oral cavity**
  Tongue thrusting/Thumb-sucking/Mouth-breathing/Nail-biting/Lip-biting/Bruxism/Others

- **Dietary habits:**
  Sugar consumption: Type: Fermentable/Less fermentable/Solid/Liquid/Sticky/Non-sticky Frequency:
  With/in-between meals:

Last visit to the dentist
Treatment record

EXAMINATION

General Physical Examination

- **General examination**
  Built and nourishment:
  Gait:
  Posture:
  Height:
  Weight:
- **Vital signs**
  BP:
  Pulse:
  Resp. rate
  Temperature:
- **Signs of anemia**: Pallor/Koilonychia/Angular stomatitis
- **Signs of cyanosis**: Tongue/Nailbed/Ear lobule
- **Eyes:**
  Sclera:
  Conjunctiva:
  Pupillary reflex:
- **Nose:** Polyp/Discharge/Swelling/DNS/Epistaxis
- **Extremities:**
  Upper limbs: Swelling/Pigmentation/Clubbing/Edema
  Lower limbs: Swelling/Pigmentation/Clubbing/Edema
- **Nails:** Color/Shape/Brittleness/Ridges
- **Skin:** Pallor/Jaundice/Cyanosis/Other findings

Extraoral Examination

Symmetry:

TMJ: *Clicking*:
Jaw deviations: Right/Left
Tenderness: Present/Absent
Trismus: Present/Absent
Swelling:

Lymph nodes:
- Submandibular
- Submental
- Pre-auricular
- Post-auricular
- Occipital

- *Cervical*: Deep superficial
- Clavicular
- Axillary
- Inguinal

Intraoral Examination

Soft tissue:

Lip:
Cheeks:
Tongue: Dorsum:
Ventral:
Lateral borders:
Movements:
Buccal mucosa:
Labial mucosa:
Vestibule:
Floor of Mouth:
Palate: Soft/Hard
Alveolar mucosa:
Orifices of Salivary Ducts:
Tonsillar Pillars:
Frenum:

Hard tissue:

Dentition: Permanent Mixed Deciduous
Teeth present:
Over retained:
Supernumerary:
Missing and reason for loss:
Root stumps:
Caries:
Restorations:
Prosthesis: Fixed/Removable/Implant
Enamel Hypoplasia:
Fluorosis:
Wasting disease: Attrition/Abrasion/Erosion/Abfraction
Occlusion:
Malformed/Malposed:
Any other anomaly:
Deposits: Stains-Plaque/Calculus-
Periodontal findings:
Gingiva: Enlargement:
Recession:
Color:
Shape:
Surface texture:

Consistency:
Bleeding on Probing:
Interdental Papillae:
Pockets: Generalized/Localized
Irritation from partial dentures:
Overhangs, if any:
Dentures: Retention:
Stability:
Vertical height: Increased/Decreased

Examination of Specific Lesion in Detail

Swelling

Extraoral

Inspection

- Site
- Shape
- Extent
- Surface texture
- Color
- Number
- Edge
- Overlying skin
- Surrounding skin
- Pulsation
- Limitation of Movements
- Sinus/Fistula/Discharge

Palpation

- Confirm inspector findings
- Temperature
- Tenderness
- Consistency
- Fixity to underlying structures: Yes/No
- Fixity to overlying structures: Yes/No
- Fluctuation: Yes/No
- Translucency: Yes/No
- Compressibility: Yes/No
- Pulsation: Yes/No
- Blanching: Yes/No

Auscultation: Yes/No

Intraoral

Inspection

- Site
- Size

- Shape
- Surface texture
- Color
- Number
- Edge
- Pulsation
- Limitation of Movements
- Sinus/Fistula/Discharge

Palpation

- Confirm inspector findings
- Temperature
- Tenderness
- Consistency
- Fixity to deeper structures:
- Fluctuation:
- Translucency: Yes/No
- Compressibility: Yes/No
- Pulsation: Yes/No
- Fixity to overlying tissue: Yes/No

Auscultation: Yes/No

Ulcer

Extraoral

Inspection:

- Size, shape and extent
- Site
- Color
- Edge: Undermined/Punched out/Sloping/Raised/Pearly wide beaded/Rolled out/Everted
- Floor
- Discharge
- Surrounding area

Palpation:

- Tenderness
- Edge
- Base
- Depth
- Bleeding: Yes/No
- Relation to deeper structures: Yes/No
- Surrounding area
- Whole area

Intraoral

Inspection:

- Size and shape
- Number
- Position
- Edge: Undermined/Punched out/Sloping/Raised/Pearly wide beaded/Rolled out/Everted
- Floor
- Discharge
- Surrounding area
- Whole area

Palpation:

- Tenderness
- Edge
- Base
- Depth
- Bleeding: Yes/No
- Relation to deeper structures: Yes/No

Provisional diagnosis:

Differential diagnosis:

Investigations

- **Blood:** CBC- Hb%/Hematocrit/RBC/WBC
  DC, BT, PT, PTT
  ESR, GTT, Calcium, Phosphorus
  Blood Sugar: Fasting
  Postprandial
  Serum Enzyme Level: Alkaline Phosphatase, SGOT/SGPT, LDH/Bilirubin/Amylase/Creatinine
  Blood Urea Nitrogen
  Creatinine Phosphokinase
  Others:
- **Urine:**
  Color, Appearance, Specific Gravity:
  pH:
  Protein:
  Glucose:
  Ketones, Bilirubin, Bence Jones:
  Blood:
- **Radiographic investigation**

  Intraoral:
  IOPA
  Bitewing
  Occlusal

Extraoral:

OPG
Lateral oblique/PA view
Any other
Chest
Extremities

- **Special investigations**
  CT Scan/Tomography/Arthrograms/Scintigraph/Ultrasound/MRI/Xerradiography
- **Vitality tests:** Thermal Heat
  Electric Pulp Testing
- **Biopsy**
  Exfoliative Cytology
  Edge Biopsy
  Incisional
  Wedge Biopsy
  Excisional
  FNAC
  Punch Biopsy
- **Culture sensitivity**
- **Immunological tests**
  ELISA
  Paul-Bunnel Test
  Radioimmune Assay
  RHF Test
  ANA
  Western Blot Test
  Others
- **Smear examination**

Final diagnosis:

Treatment plan:

Drugs prescribed:

Prognosis:

Follow-up:

Date	Findings	Drugs prescribed	Next Appointment

Summary

Annexure

CAUSES OF A BURNING SENSATION IN THE MOUTH	
Local causes	*Systemic causes*
• Erythema migraines (Geographical tongue) • Lichen planus • Candidosis • Denture problems	• Psychogenic • Cancerophobia • Depression • Anxiety states • Hypochondriasis • Deficiency of: Vitamin B, especially B_{12}, Folate and Iron • Dry mouth • Diabetes • Drugs

CAUSES OF DRY MOUTH	
Iatrogenic	*Disease*
• Drugs • Irradiation • Graft versus host disease	• Dehydration, psychogenic, salivary gland disease, Sjögren's syndrome, sarcoidosis, salivary aplasia

DRUGS ASSOCIATED WITH DRY MOUTH	
Drugs which directly damage the salivary glands	Cytotoxic drugs
Drugs with anticholinergic activity	Anticholinergic agents such as atropine, and hyoscine Antireflux agents, e.g. proton-pump inhibitors Psychoactive agents with anticholinergic activities such as antidepressants including tricyclic, selective serotonin re-uptake inhibitors, lithium and others. Phenothiazines, benzodiazepines, opioids, antihistamines, bupropion
Drugs acting on sympathetic system	Drugs with sympathomimetic activity, e.g. ephedrine, antihypertensives; alpha 1 antagonists and alpha 2 agonists may reduce salivary flow. Beta-blockers also change salivary protein levels.
Drugs which deplete fluid	Diuretics

CAUSES OF HALITOSIS	
Oral infections	*Systemic disease*
• Starvation • Dry mouth • *Habits*: Smoking, alcohol and some drugs Some foods	• Diabetic ketosis, hepatic failure, respiratory disease, psychogenic factors, gastrointestinal disease, renal failure, trimethylaminuria,

CAUSES OF ORAL BROWN OR BLACK HYPERPIGMENTATION		
Localized	*Multiple or Generalized*	
• Amalgam, graphite, carbon, dyes, inks or other tattoos • Ephelis (Freckle) • Epithelioid angiomatosis • Kaposi's sarcoma • Malignant melanoma • Melanoacanthoma • Melanotic macules • Nevus • Pigmented neuroectodermal tumor • Verruciform xanthoma	**Genetic** • Racial, Carney syndrome, complex of myxomas, spotty pigmentation and endocrine overactivity, Laugier-Hunziker syndrome, Lentiginosis profuse, Leopard syndrome, Peutz-Jeghers syndrome **Drugs** • ACTH, Amiodarone, Antimalarials, Betel, Busulphan, Chlorpromazine, Clofazamine, contraceptive pill, Ketoconazole, Menthol, Metals (bismuth, mercury, silver, gold, arsenic, copper, chromium, cobalt, manganese) Methyldopa, Minocycline, Phenothiazines, Smoking, Zidovudine	**Endocrine** • Addison's disease, Albright's syndrome, Nelson's syndrome, Pregnancy **Post-inflammatory** **Others** • Gaucher's disease • Generalized neurofibromatosis Hemochromatosis • HIV disease • Incontinentia pigmenti • Thalassemia • Whipple's disease • Wilson's disease

COMMON CAUSES OF WHITE LESIONS

Local causes
- Materia alba (Debris from poor oral hygiene)
- Keratosis
- Frictional keratosis (Cheek/lip-biting)
- Smoker's keratosis
- Snuff-Dipper's keratosis
- Burns
- Grafts
- Scars
- Furred or hairy tongue

Neoplastic and possibly preneoplastic
- Leukoplakia
- Keratosis
- Carcinoma

Inflammatory

Infective
- Candidiasis
- Hairy leukoplakia
- Syphilitic mucous patches and keratosis
- Koplik's spots (Measles)
- Some papillomas
- Reiter's disease
- Koilocytic dysplasia (Papillomavirus)

Non-infective
- Lichen planus
- Lupus erythematosus

Congenital
- Leukoedema
- Fordyce's spots
- Inherited dyskeratosis
- White sponge nevus
- Focal palmoplantar and oral mucosa hyperkeratosis syndrome
- Darier's disease
- Pachyonychia congenita
- Dyskeratosis congenita

COMMON CAUSES OF RED LESIONS

Localized

Inflammatory lesions
- Geographic tongue, candidiasis, lichen planus, drugs

Reactive lesions
- Pyogenic granulomas
- Peripheral giant cell granulomas

Atrophic lesions
- Geographic tongue
- Lichen planus
- Lupus erythematosus
- Erythroplasia
- Avitaminosis B_{12}

Purpura: Trauma, thrombocytopenia

Vascular: Telangiectases (Hereditary hemorrhagic telangiectasia or scleroderma or post-irradiation angiomas)

Neoplasms: Squamous carcinoma, Kaposi's sarcoma, Giant cell tumor, Wegener's granulomatosis

Generalized

Inflammatory lesions
- Most red lesions are inflammatory, usually geographic tongue (Erythema migrans)

Viral infections (e.g. herpes simplex stomatitis)

Fungal infections: Candidiasis-denture-related stomatitis, median rhomboid glossitis and acute oral candidiasis

Bacterial infections
- Cancer treatment-related mucositis; common after irradiation of tumors of the head and neck, or chemotherapy e.g. for leukemia
- Immunological reactions such as lichen planus, plasma cell gingivostomatitis, granulomatous disorders (Sarcoidosis, Crohn's disease, orofacial granulomatosis), amyloidosis, and graft versus host disease

Avitaminosis B or iron deficiency or folate deficiency

MAIN CAUSES OF ORAL ULCERS

Local causes
- Trauma, appliances, iatrogenic, non-accidental injury, self-inflicted, sharp teeth or restorations, burns, chemical, cold, electric, heat, radiation

Recurrent aphthae

Infections
- Acute narcotizing gingivitis
- Chickenpox
- Deep mycoses
- Hand, foot and mouth disease
- Herpangina
- Herpetic stomatitis
- HIV
- Infectious mononucleosis
- Syphilis
- Tuberculosis

Drugs
- Cytotoxic drugs, nicorandil, NSAIDs and many others

Hematological disorders
- Anemia, gammopathies, Hematinic deficiencies, Leukemia and myelodysplastic syndrome, Neutropenia and other white cell dyscrasias

Malignant neoplasms

Oral
- Encroaching from antrum
- Systemic disease
- Mucocutaneous disease
- Behçet's syndrome
- Chronic ulcerative stomatitis
- Epidermolysis bullosa
- Erythema multiforme
- Lichen planus
- Pemphigus vulgaris
- Sub-epithelial immune blistering diseases (Pemphigoid and variants, dermatitis herpetiformis, linear IgA disease)

Gastrointestinal disease
- Celiac disease, Crohn's disease, Ulcerative colitis

Miscellaneous uncommon diseases
- Eosinophilic ulcer
- Giant cell arteritis
- Hypereosinophilic syndrome
- Lupus erythematosus
- Narcotizing sialometaplasia
- Periarteritis nodosa
- Reiter's syndrome and Sweet's syndrome
- Wegener's granulomatosis

UNCOMMON SUB-EPITHELIAL VESICULOBULLOUS DISORDERS

- Pemphigoid variants
- Erythema multiforme
- Acquired epidermolysis bullosa (EBA)
- Toxic epidermal necrolysis (TEN)
- Chronic bullous dermatosis of childhood dermatitis herpetiformis
- Linear IgA disease

CLASSIFICATION OF THE NECK NODES ACCORDING TO THE ANATOMY

Upper horizontal chain of nodes	*Lateral cervical nodes*	*Anterior cervical nodes*
Submental Submandibular Parotid Postauricular Occipital	Superficial external jugular group Deep group • Internal jugular group (Upper, middle and lower) • Spinal accessory chain • Transverse cervical chain	Anterior jugular chain Juxtavisceral chain • Prelaryngeal • Pretracheal • Paratracheal

CLASSIFICATION OF THE NECK NODES ACCORDING TO THE LEVELS		
Levels	*Nodes*	*Location*
Level I	Submental (IA)	In the submental triangle, i.e. between the right and left anterior bellies of the diagastric and the hyoid.
	Submandibular (IB)	Lies between the anterior and posterior bellies of the diagastric and the body the mandible.
Level II	Upper jugular	Upper third of the jugular vein, i.e. between the skull base above, and the level of the hyoid bone below.
Level III	Middle jugular	Along the middle third of jugular vein, from the level of the hyoid bone above to the cricoid cartilage below.
Level IV	Lower jugular	Along the middle third of the jugular vein, from upper border of the cricoid cartilage to the clavicle.
Level V	Posterior triangle group	In the posterior triangle, i.e. posterior border of sternocleidomastoid (anteriorly), the trapezius (posteriorly) and the clavicle below. Includes lymph nodes of the spinal accessory chain, transverse cervical nodes and the supraclavicular nodes.
Level VI	Anterior compartment nodes	Between the medial borders of the sterno-cleidomastoid muscles (or the carotid sheath) on each side, hyoid bone above and the suprasternal notch below. Includes prelaryngeal, pretracheal, paratracheal nodes.
Level VII	Nodes of upper mediastinum	Below the suprasternal notch

LYMPHATIC DRAINAGE OF ORAL CAVITY	
Gingiva	Maxillary—deep cervical nodes, Mandibular—submandibular nodes
Hard palate	Superior deep cervical
Soft palate	Superior deep cervical and retropharyngeal nodes
Cheek	Submandibular nodes
Floor of mouth	Anterior—Upper deep cervical nodes Posterior—Submandibular and superior deep cervical nodes
Teeth	Maxillary—Deep cervical nodes Mandibular—submandibular, submental
Tonsils	Superior deep cervical nodes
Tongue	Anterior 2/3rd—submental, submandibular and deep cervical nodes Posterior 1/3rd—jugulodiagastric and jugulomylohyoid nodes
Lips	Upper lip and lower lip, lateral part—submandibular nodes, lower lip—submental nodes

EVALUATION OF SUSPECTED CAUSES OF LYMPHADENOPATHY		
Disorder	*Associated features*	*Investigations*
• HIV infection	• "Flu-like" illness, rash	• ELISA, Western blot
• Mononucleosis-type syndromes	• Fatigue, malaise, fever, atypical lymphocytosis	• Mono spot, Paul-Bunnel test
• Cat-scratch disease	• Fever in one third of patients; axillary nodes	• Usually clinical criteria; biopsy, if necessary
• Tuberculosis lymphadenitis	• Painless, matted nodes	• PPD, biopsy
• Cytomegalovirus	• Often mild symptoms; patients may have hepatitis	• IgM CMV antibody, viral culture of urine or blood
• Toxoplasmosis	• 80–90% of patients are asymptomatic	• IgM toxoplasma antibody
• Lymphoma	• Fever, night sweats, weight loss in 20–30% of patients	• Biopsy
• Sarcoidosis	• Hilar node, skin lesion, dyspnea	• Biopsy
• Leukemia	• Blood dyscrasias, bruising	• Blood smear, bone marrow
• Kawasaki disease	• Fever, conjunctivitis, rash, mucous membrane lesions	• Clinical criteria
• Lupus erythematosus	• Arthritis, rash, serositis, renal, neurologic, hematologic disorders	• Clinical criteria, antinuclear antibodies, complement levels
• Streptococcal pharyngitis	• Fever, pharyngeal exudates,	• Throat culture
• Hepatitis B	• Fever, nausea, vomiting, icterus	• Liver function tests, HBsAg

CONDITIONS WHICH MAY PRESENT AS LUMPS OR SWELLINGS IN THE ORAL CAVITY	
Normal anatomy	Pterygoid hamulus, Parotid papillae, lingual papillae (foliate and circumvallate)
Developmental	Unerupted teeth, odontogenic cysts, eruption cysts, developmental cysts (e.g. thyroglossal, dermoid), lymphangioma, hemangioma, tori, hereditary gingival fibromatosis, lingual thyroid
Inflammatory	Abscess, cellulitis, cysts, insect bites, sialadenitis, pyogenic granuloma, orofacial granulomatosis, crohn's disease, sarcoidosis, chronic granulomatous disorders
Traumatic	Denture granulomata, epulis, fibroepithelial polyp, mucocele, hematoma, surgical emphysema
Neoplasms	Carcinoma, leukemia, lymphoma, myeloma
Odontogenic tumors	Minor salivary glands, others
Fibro-osseous	Cherubism, fibrous dysplasia, Paget's disease

Contd...

Contd...

Hormonal	Pregnancy epulis/gingivitis, oral contraceptive pill gingivitis
Metabolic	Amyloidosis, other deposits
Drugs	Phenytoin, calcium-channel blockers, cyclosporin
Allergic	Angioedema
Infective	HPV

CAUSES OF SALIVARY GLAND SWELLING	
Inflammatory	Mumps Ascending sialadenitis Recurrent parotitis HIV parotitis Other infections (e.g. tuberculosis) Sjögren's syndrome Sarcoidosis
Neoplasms	Mainly pleomorphic salivary adenoma, but also monomorphic adenomas
Duct obstruction	e.g. Calculus
Sialosis	Usually caused by autonomic dysfunction in starvation, bulimia, diabetes, or alcoholic cirrhosis
Deposits rarely	Amyloidosis and hemochromatosis
Drugs rarely	Chlorhexidine, methyldopa, phenylbutazone, iodine compounds, thiouracil, catecholamines, sulfonamides, phenothiazines and protease inhibitors

ORAL MALIGNANT NEOPLASMS

Common oral squamous cell carcinoma

Cancers of the oral cavity are classified according to site:

- Lip
- Tongue
- Gum
- Floor of the mouth
- Unspecified parts of the mouth

Less common

- Kaposi's sarcoma
- Lymphoma
- Malignant melanoma
- Maxillary antral carcinoma (or other neoplasms)
- Metastatic neoplasms (Breast, lung, kidney, stomach, liver)
- Neoplasms of bone and connective tissue

Odontogenic tumors

Salivary gland tumors

CHARACTERISTIC FEATURES OF POTENTIAL MALIGNANT CONDITIONS OF THE ORAL CAVITY		
Lesion	*Etiology*	*Features*
• Erythroplakia	• Tobacco/alcohol	• Flat red plaque
• Leukoplakia	• Tobacco/alcohol	• White or speckled plaque
• Proliferative verrucous leukoplakia	• Tobacco/alcohol/human papillomavirus (HPV)	• White or speckled or nodular plaque
• Sublingual keratosis	• Tobacco/alcohol	• White plaque
• Actinic cheilitis	• Sunlight	• White plaque/erosions
• Lichen planus	• Idiopathic	• White plaque/erosions/ red lesions
• Submucous fibrosis	• Areca nut	• Immobile mucosa
• Discoid lupus erythematosus	• Idiopathic	• White plaque/erosions
• Chronic candidosis	• Candida albicans	• White or speckled plaque
• Syphilitic leukoplakia	• Syphilis	• White plaque
• Atypia in immunocompromised patients	• Papillomavirus	• White or speckled plaque
• Dyskeratosis congenita	• Genetic	• White plaques
• Patterson-Kelly syndrome (Sideropenic dysphagia; Plummer–Vinson syndrome)	• Iron deficiency	• Postcricoid web

TNM CLASSIFICATION OF MALIGNANT NEOPLASM	
Primary tumor size (T)	
Tx	No available information
T0	No evidence of primary tumor
Tis	Only carcinoma *in situ*
T1, T2, T3, T4	Increasing size of tumor*
Regional lymph node involvement (N)	
Nx	Nodes could not or were not assessed
N0	No clinically positive nodes
N1	Single clinically positive ipsilateral node less than 3 cm in diameter
N2	Single clinically positive ipsilateral node 3–6 cm in diameter, or multiple clinically positive homolateral nodes, none more than 6 cm in diameter
N2a	Single clinically positive ipsilateral node 3–6 cm in diameter
N2b	Multiple clinically positive ipsilateral nodes, none more than 6 cm in diameter
N3	Massive ipsilateral node(s), bilateral nodes, or contralateral node(s)

Contd...

Contd...

N3a	Clinically positive ipsilateral node(s), one more than 6 cm in diameter
N3b	Bilateral clinically positive nodes
N3c	Contralateral clinically positive node(s)
Involvement by distant metastases(M)	
Mx	Distant metastasis was not assessed
M0	No evidence of distant metastasis
M1, M2, M3	Distant metastasis is present. Increasing degrees of metastatic involvement, including distant nodes

* T1 maximum diameter 2 cm; T2 maximum diameter of 4 cm; T3 maximum diameter over 4 cm. T4 massive tumor greater than 4 cm diameter, with involvement of antrum, pterygoid muscles, base of tongue or skin.

LENGTH AND DIAMETER OF THE NEEDLES USED FOR FNAC

Gauze	*Available length*	*Outside diameter*	*Inside diameter*
20	25, 38, 76	0.89	0.58
22	19, 25, 38	0.71	0.41
23	6, 19, 25	0.64	0.33
25	16, 25, 32, 51, 88	0.51	0.25
27	13, 19, 28	0.41	0.20

NORMAL CONCENTRATION OF CONSTITUENTS OF SALIVA (MG/100 ML) (JENKIN'S 4TH EDN)

Organic and inorganic	*Whole saliva*		*Parotid saliva*		*Submandibular saliva*	
constituents	*Resting*	*Stimulated*	*Resting*	*Stimulated*	*Resting*	*Stimulated*
Protein	140–640	170–420	100	100–300	30–80	30–150
Amylase	38	-	60	120	25	-
Lysozyme	22	0.4–62	-	0.5–8	-	0.5–4.2
IgA	19	-	-	1.7–6.3	1.6	-
IgG	1.4	-	-	0–0.1	-	-
IgM	0.2	-	-	0.4	-	-
Glucose	1.0	0.5–3.0	1	0.2	-	-
Ammonia	-	1–12	0.9	0.3	0.9	0.08
Urea	12–70	0.6–30	26	10–16	10.5	20
Uric acid	0.5–3.0	1–22	4	7	3.3	1.3
Creatinine	0.05–0.2	-	-	-	-	-
Cholesterol	2.5–50	-	-	1–5	-	2.0
Na	0–20	60	12–72	115–2600	6	20–120

Contd...

Contd...

Organic and inorganic constituents	*Whole saliva*		*Parotid saliva*		*Submandibular saliva*	
	Resting	*Stimulated*	*Resting*	*Stimulated*	*Resting*	*Stimulated*
K	60–100	80	100–320	48–125	60	20–80
Ca	2.2–11.3	6	2-8	2–10	6	6–12
Mg	-	-	0.2–1.5	0.02–0.80	0.17	0.08
Cl	50	100	60–140	35–175	42	35–140
HCO_3	-	-	3–30	30–360	13	18–200
P	6.1–71	12	12–60	6–15	15	0.6–42

VERTICAL ANGULATIONS AND CENTERING POINT FOR BISECTING ANGLE TECHNIQUE

Teeth	*Vertical angulations*	*Centering point*
Maxillary incisors	+45° to +50°	Tip of nose
Maxillary canines	+50° to +55°	Ala of nose
Maxillary premolars	+30° to +35°	Meeting point of perpendicular drawn from midpoint of infraorbital margin to ala tragus line
Maxillary molars	+20° to +25°	Meeting point of perpendicular drawn from outer canthus of eye to ala tragus line
Mandibular incisors	–15° to –20°	Symphysis menti
Mandibular canines	–20° to –25°	Meeting point of perpendicular drawn from ala of nose to the inferior border of mandible
Mandibular premolars	–10° to –15°	Meeting point of perpendicular drawn from midpoint of infraorbital margin to the inferior border of mandible
Mandibular molars	–5° to –10°	Meeting point of perpendicular drawn from outer canthus of eye to the inferior border of mandible

DIRECTION OF CENTRAL RAY FOR MAXILLARY AND MANDIBULAR OCCLUSAL PROJECTIONS

Projection	*Direction of central ray*
Anterior maxillary	Central ray oriented through tip of nose towards middle of the film with vertical angulation of +45° and horizontal angulation of 0°
Cross-sectional maxillary	Central ray oriented through bridge of nose towards the middle of film with vertical angulation of +65° and horizontal angulation of 0°
Lateral maxillary	Central ray oriented through a point 2 cm below the lateral canthus of eye directed towards center of the film with vertical angulation of +60° and horizontal angulation of 0°

Contd...

Contd...

Projection	*Direction of central ray*
Anterior mandibular	Central ray oriented with –10° angulation through the point of the chin
Cross-sectional mandibular	Central ray directed to the midline through the floor of the mouth approximately 3 cm below the chin, at right angle to the center of the film
Lateral mandibular	Central ray directed perpendicular to the center of the film through a point beneath the chin, approximately 3 cm posterior and 3 cm lateral to the midline

PROBLEMS ENCOUNTERED WHILE RECORDING HISTORY OF GERIATRIC PATIENTS

Hearing loss	• Common in the elderly • May be helped by hearing aid • Important to speak clearly and slowly • Face the patient and avoid extraneous sound • If necessary, write questions in bold letters
Visual handicap	• Cataracts, glaucoma and macular degeneration are common in the elderly • Ensure the room is well lit • Engage an assistant or carer to help patients move in and out of the consulting room and examination area
Dementia	• Often occurs in patients who appear physically fit • Forgetfulness, repetition and inappropriate answers characterize responses • Family members, friends and carers often note the development of dementia
Important aspects of a history from elderly patients include	• Domestic environment and general living conditions • Family support structures • Economic status and pension provision • Provision of community and social services • Mobility (at home and in the local environment) • Detailed drug history and compliance

RECOMMENDED DRUGS FOR MEDICAL EMERGENCIES

- Adrenaline 1 mL ampules of 1 : 1000 solution for intramuscular (IM) injection
- Aspirin 300 mg dispersible tablets
- Glucagon for IM injection of 1 mg
- Glyceryl trinitrate (GTN) spray, 400 µg per metered dose
- Midazolam buccal liquid, 10 mg/mL, or midazolam injection (as hydrochloride) 5 mg/mL, 2 mL ampules, for topical buccal administration
- Oral glucose (Alternative forms, including non-diet fizzy drinks, glucose gel, powdered glucose and sugar lumps)
- Oxygen cylinder, 2 size D or 2 size CD or one size E
- Salbutamol inhaler, 100 µg/actuation

SUPPLEMENTAL STEROID COVER ACCORDING TO CURRENT DAILY DOSE	
Current daily dose of prednisolone	*Supplementary steroid cover required*
10 mg	Assume normal HPA response. Usual preoperative steroids, no supplemental steroid cover required.
> 10 mg	Simple surgery under LA (e.g. single extraction, gingivectomy): usual preoperative steroids, no supplemental steroid cover required. *Minor surgery (e.g. surgical extractions or multiple extraction)*: Usual preoperative steroids; 25 mg hydrocortisone IV before surgery/at induction of anesthesia. Moderate surgery (e.g. mandible/zygoma); usual preoperative steroids 25 mg hydrocortisone at induction of anesthesia plus 100 mg IV over 24 hours. Major surgery (e.g. head and neck/orthographic surgery): Usual preoperative steroids 25 mg hydrocortisone IV plus 100 mg/day IV for 48–72 hours. Patients who have not received steroids for more than 3 months require no perioperative supplementation.

CLINICAL CHEMISTRY OF BODY FLUIDS	
Normal Hematologic Values	
Component	*Conventional values*
Hemoglobin	
Infants	15–25 g/dL
Children (up to 1 year)	11–14 g/dL
Children (10–12 years)	11.5–14.5 g/dL
Men	14–18 g/dL
Women	12–16 g/dL
Pregnant women	11–14 g/dL
Packed cell volume (Hemotocrit)	
At Birth	54%
2 months	42%
1–2 years	36%
4 years	37%
8 years	39%
12 years	40%
Male	40–54%
Female	36–48%
Erythrocyte sedimentation rate (ESR)	
In newborn	0–5 mm
Children	3–10 mm
Male	0–15 mm
Female	0–20 mm
Mean cell volume (MCV)	77–93 fL
Mean corpuscular hemoglobin (MCH)	27–32 pg
Mean corpuscular hemoglobin concentration (MCHC)	30–35 g/dL

Contd...

Contd...

Component	*Conventional values*
Red blood cell count	
At birth	6.5–7.5 million/mm^3
Males	4.5–6.5 million/mm^3
Females	3.8–5.8 million/mm^3
Total leukocyte count (TLC)	
At birth	10,000–25,000/cumm
1-3 years	6,000–18,000/cumm
4-7 years	6,000–15,000/cumm
8-12 years	4,500–13,500/cumm
Adults	4,000–11,000/cumm
Differential leukocyte count (DLC)	
Neutrophils	40–75% (3000–7000/cumm)
Eosinophils	1–6% (40–400/cumm)
Basophils	<1% (0–100/cumm)
Lymphocytes	20–45% (1500–4000/cumm)
Monocytes	2–8% (200–800/cumm)
Absolute eosinophil count	40–400 cells/cumm
Reticulocyte count	
Infants	0.8–4%
Adults	0.8–2.5%
Platelet count	1.5–4 lac/cumm
Bleeding time (BT)	1–5 min (Duke's method) 2–8 min (Ivy's method)
Clotting time (CT)	1–7 min (Capillary tube method) 5–10 min (Lee and White method) 2.5–5 min (Kruse and Moses method)
Prothrombin time (PT)	10–15 sec (Quick's one stage method)
Partial thromboplastin time (PTT)	30–50 sec
Activated partial thromboplastin Time (aPTT)	15–35 sec
Thrombin time (TT)	<20 seconds
Serum iron	55–185 µgm/cumm
Total iron binding capacity	250–425 µgm/cumm
Serum fibrinogen	200–400 mg/dL
General Chemistry	
Acetone	0.3–2.0 mg%
Alanine aminotransferase (ALT)	7–56 U/L
Albumin	3.5–5.0 gm/dL
Albumin (Newborn)	2.9–5.5 gm/dL
Albumin (Child)	3.8–5.4 gm/dL
Alkaline phosphatase	32–110 U/L
Anion gap	5–16 mEq/L
Ammonia	11–35 µmol/L
Amylase	50–150 U/dL
Anti-streptolysin O titer (ASO) (Adult)	<125

Contd...

Contd...

Component	*Conventional values*
Anti-streptolysin O Titer (ASO) (Child)	<250
AST, SGOT (Male)	7–21 U/L
AST, SGOT (Female)	6–18 U/L
Bilirubin (Direct)	0.0–0.4 mg/dL
Bilirubin (Indirect)	Total minus direct
Bilirubin (Total)	0.2–1.4 mg/dL
BUN	6–23 mg/dL
Calcium (Total)	8–11 mg/dL
Carbon dioxide	21–34 mEq/L
Carbon monoxide	Symptoms at greater than or equal to 10% saturation
Chloride	96–112 mEq/L
CK-MM	96–100%
CK-BB	0%
Cortisol (8 am)	5–25 gm/dL
Cortisol (8 am)	2–9 gm/dL
Creatine (Male)	0.2–0.6 mg/dL
Creatine (Female)	0.6–1.0 mg/dL
Creatinine	0.6–1.5 mg/dL
Creatinine (Newborn)	0.3–0.7 mg/dL
Creatinine (Child)	0.3–1.0 mg/dL
Creatinine Kinase Isoenzyme, MB	0–121 U/L
Creatinine Phosphokinase (CPK)	24–195 U/L
Ethanol	0 mg%; Coma: greater than or equal to 400–500 mg%
Ferritin (Male)	18–250 ng/mL
Ferritin (Female)	12–160 ng/mL
Folate	3.6–20 ng/mL
Folic acid	2.0–21 ng/mL
Gamma GT	8–78 U/L
Gamma-glutamyl transferase (GGT) (Male)	1–94 U/L
Gamma-glutamyl transferase (GGT) (Female)	1–70 U/L
Glucose	70–110 mg/dL (Diuresis greater than or equal to 180 mg/dL)
Growth hormone (Male)	0–4 ng/mL
Growth hormone (Female)	0–18 ng/mL
IGF-1 (male)	54–329 ng/mL
IGF-1 (female)	142–329 ng/mL
HDL (Male)	25–65 mg/dL
HDL (Female)	38–94 mg/dL
Insulin	0–180 pmol/L
Iron	52–169 µg/dL
Iron-binding capacity	246–455 µg/dL
Lactic acid	0.4–2.3 mEq/L
Lactate	0.3–2.3 mEq/L
Lipase	10–140 U/L

Contd...

Contd...

Component	*Conventional values*
Magnesium	1.5–2.5 mg/dL
Osmolarity	276–295 mOsm/kg
Parathyroid hormone	12–68 pg/mL
Phosphorus	2.2–4.8 mg/dL
Potassium	3.5–5.5 mEq/L
Protein (Total)	6.0–9.0 gm/dL
SGPT	8–32 U/L
Sodium	135–148 mEq/L
T3	0.8–1.1 μg/dL
Thyroglobulin	Less than 55 ng/mL
Thyroxine (T4) total	5–13 μg/dL
Thyroxine-binding globulin (TBG)	12–30 mg/L
Free thyroxine (T4 Free)	0.8–1.5 ng/dL
Total protein	5–9 gm/dL
Total serum iron (Male)	76–198 μg/dL
Total serum iron (Female)	26–170 μg/dL
Transferrin	204–360 mg/dL
TSH	Less than 9 μU/mL
Urea nitrogen (BUN)	7–25 mg/dL
Uric acid (Male)	3.5–7.7 mg/dL
Uric acid (Female)	2.5–6.6 mg/dL
Lipid Profile	
Cholesterol (total)	Less than 200 mg/dL desirable
Cholesterol (HDL)	30–75 mg/dL
Cholesterol (LDL)	Less than 130 mg/dL desirable
Triglycerides (Male)	Greater than 40–170 mg/dL
Triglycerides (Female)	Greater than 35–135 mg/dL
Normal Urine Values	
Color	Straw
Specific gravity	1.003–1.040
pH	4.6–8.0
Na	10–40 mEq/L
K	Less than 8 mEq/L
Cl	Less than 8 mEq/L
Protein	1–15 mg/dL
Osmolality	80–1300 mOsm/L
24-hour Urine Analysis	
Amylase	250–1100 IU/24 hr
Calcium	100–250 mg/24 hr
Chloride	110–250 mEq/24 hr
Creatinine	1–2 g/24 hr
Creatine clearance (Male)	100–140 mL/min
Creatine clearance (Male)	16–26 mg/kg/24 hr
Creatine clearance (Female)	80–130 mL/min

Contd...

Contd…

Component	*Conventional values*
Creatine clearance (Female)	10–20 mg/kg/24 hr
Magnesium	6–9 mEq/24 hr
Osmolality	450–900 mOsm/kg
Phosphorus	0.9–1.3 g/24 hr
Potassium	35–85 mEq/24 hr
Protein	0–150 mg/24 hr
Sodium	30–280 mEq/24 hr
Urea nitrogen	10–22 gm/24 hr
Uric acid	240–755 mg/24 hr
Cerebral Spinal Fluid	
Appearance	Clear
Glucose	40–85 mg/dL
Osmolality	290–298 mOsm/L
Pressure	70–180 mm/H_2O
Protein	15–45 mg/dL
Total cell count	0–5 cells
WBCs	0–6/μL
Cardiac Markers	
Troponin I	0–0.1 ng/mL (onset: 4–6 hrs, peak: 12–24 h, return to normal: 4-7 days)
Troponin T	0–0.2 ng/mL (onset: 3–4 hr, peak: 10–24 hrs, return to normal: 10-14 days)
Myoglobin (Male)	10–95 ng/mL (onset: 1–3 hrs, peak: 6–10 hrs, return to normal: 12–24 hr)
Myoglobin (Female)	10–65 ng/mL (onset: 1–3 hr, peak: 6–10 hrs, return to normal: 12–24 hr)
Troponin I	0–0.1 ng/mL (onset: 4–6 hrs, peak: 12–24 hr, return to normal: 4–7 days)
Creatinine kinase index (CK-Index)	0–3
Creatinine kinase-MB (CK-MB)	0–3 ng/mL
Total creatinine kinase	38–120 ng/mL

VITAL SIGNS AND BODY MASS INDEX	
Blood Pressure (Systolic/Diastolic)	
At physicians office (Average 5 measurements)	<140/90 mm Hg
Ambulatory BP	<135/85 mm Hg
With diabetes	<130/80 mm Hg
Heart Rate (HR) or Pulse	
Bradycardia	<60 beats per minute
Normal	60–80
Tachycardia	>100

Contd…

Contd…

Respiration Rate (RR)	
Bradypnea	<12 breaths per minute
Normal (Eupnea)	12–18
Tachypnea	>18
Body Temperature	
Fever	>37.5°C
Normal	36.5–37.5°C (Approximate)
Hypothermia	<35.0°C
Body Mass Index (BMI)	
Underweight	<18.5 kg/m^2
Normal (Health Canada 2012)	18.5–24.9 (Caucasian)
Overweight	25.0–29.9
Obesity class I	30.0–34.9
Obesity class II	35.0–39.9
Obesity class III (Extreme, morbid)	≥40.0

Glossary

A

Abscess: Acute or chronic localized inflammation, probably with a collection of pus, associated with tissue destruction and, frequently, swelling; usually secondary to infection.

Acute periradicular or acute apical abscess: An inflammatory reaction to pulpal infection and necrosis characterized by rapid onset, spontaneous pain, tenderness of the tooth to pressure, pus formation and eventual swelling of associated tissues. May also be known as acute periapical abscess, acute alveolar abscess, dentoalveolar abscess, phoenix abscess, recrudescent abscess, secondary apical abscess.

Abutment: A tooth or implant fixture used as a support for a prosthesis.

Abutment crown: Artificial crown also serving for the retention or support of a dental prosthesis.

Acid etching: Use of an acidic chemical substance to prepare the tooth enamel and or dentin surface to provide retention for bonding.

Adhesion: State in which two surfaces are held together by chemical or physical forces or both with or without the aid of an adhesive. Adhesion is one aspect of bonding.

Adhesive: Any substance that joins or creates close adherence of two or more surfaces. Intermediate material that causes two materials to adhere to each other.

Adjunctive: A secondary treatment in addition to the primary therapy.

Adult dentition: The permanent teeth of adulthood that either replace the primary dentition or erupt distally to the primary molars.

Allogenic: Belonging to the same species, but genetically different.

Allograft: Graft of tissue between genetically dissimilar members of the same species. Donors may be cadavers, living-related or living-unrelated individuals. It is also called allogenic graft or homograft.

Alloplastic: It refers to synthetic material often used for tissue augmentation or replacement.

Alloy: Compound combining two or more elements having properties not existing in any of the single constituent elements.

Alveolar: Referring to the bone to which a tooth is attached.

Alveoloplasty: Surgical procedure for recontoring supporting bone, sometimes in preparation for a prosthesis.

Amalgam: An alloy used in direct dental restorations. Typically composed of mercury, silver, tin and copper along with other metallic elements added to improve physical and mechanical properties.

Anatomical crown: That portion of tooth normally covered by, and including, enamel.

Ancillary: Subordinate or auxiliary to something or someone else; supplementary.

Analgesia: The diminution or elimination of pain.

Anomaly: Deviation from the normal anatomic structure, growth, development or function; an abnormality.

Anxiolysis: The diminution or elimination of anxiety.

Apex: The tip or end of the root end of the tooth.

Apexification: The process of induced root development to encourage the formation of a calcified barrier in a tooth with immature root formation or an open apex. It may involve the placement of an artificial apical barrier prior to nonsurgical endodontic obturation.

Apexogenesis: Vital pulp therapy performed to encourage continued physiological formation and development of the tooth root.

Apicoectomy: Amputation of the apex of a tooth.

Arch, dental: The curved composite structure of the natural dentition and the residual ridge, or the remains thereof, after the loss of some or all of the natural teeth.

Arthrogram: A diagnostic X-ray technique used to view bone structures following injection of a contrast medium into a joint.

Artificial crown: Restoration covering or replacing the major part, or the whole of the clinical crown of a tooth, or implant.

Autogenous graft: Taken from one part of a patient's body and transferred to another.

Avulsion: Separation of tooth from its socket due to trauma.

B

Barrier membrane: Usually a thin, sheet-like usually non-autogenous material used in various surgical regenerative procedures.

Behavior management: Techniques or therapies used to alter or control the actions of a patient who is receiving dental treatment. Examples include use of a papoose board, education or anxiety relief techniques.

Benign: The mild or non-threatening character of an illness or the non-malignant character of a neoplasm.

Bicuspid: A premolar tooth; a tooth with two cusps.

Bilateral: Occurring on, or pertaining to, both right and left sides.

Biologic materials: Agents that alter wound healing or host-tumor interaction. Such materials can include cytokines, growth factor, or vaccines, but do not include any actual hard or soft tissue graft material. These agents are added to graft material or used alone to effect acceleration of healing or regeneration in hard and soft tissue surgical procedures. Also known as biologic response modifiers.

Biopsy: Process of removing tissue for histologic evaluation.

Bitewing radiograph: Interproximal radiographic view of the coronal portion of the tooth/teeth. A form of dental radiograph that may be taken with the long axis of the image oriented either horizontally or vertically, that reveals approximately the coronal halves of the maxillary and mandibular teeth and portions of the interdental alveolar septa on the same image.

Bleaching: Process of lightening of the teeth, usually using a chemical oxidizing agent and sometimes in the presence of heat. Removal of deep seated intrinsic or acquired discolorations from crowns of vital and non-vital teeth through by the use of chemicals, sometimes in combination with the application of heat and light. Bleaching has been achieved through short- and long-term applications of pastes or solutions containing various concentrations of hydrogen peroxide and carbamide peroxide. Normally applied externally to teeth; may be used internally for endodontically treated teeth.

Bonding: Process by which two or more components are made integral by mechanical and/or chemical adhesion at their interface.

Bruxism: The parafunctional grinding of the teeth.

Buccal: Pertaining to or toward the cheek (as in the buccal surface of a posterior tooth).

C

Calculus: Hard deposit of mineralized substance adhering to crowns and/or roots of teeth or prosthetic devices.

Canal: A relatively narrow tubular passage or channel.

Cantilever extension: Part of a fixed prosthesis that extends beyond the abutment to which it is attached and has no additional support.

Caries: Commonly used term for tooth decay.

Carious lesion: A cavity caused by caries.

Case management: The monitoring and coordination of treatment rendered to patients with specific diagnoses or requiring high cost or extensive services. It may include complex treatment plans or discussion between multiple practitioners.

A process of identifying patients with special healthcare needs, developing a healthcare strategy that meets those needs, and coordinating and monitoring the care, with the ultimate goal of achieving the optimum healthcare outcome in an efficient and cost-effective manner.

Cavity: Missing tooth structure. A cavity may be due to decay, erosion or abrasion. If caused by caries; it is also referred to as carious lesion.

Cellulitis: A lesion of acute inflammation consisting of diffuse spreading purulent exudate.

Cement base: Material used under a filling to replace lost tooth structure.

Cementum: Hard connective tissue covering the outer surface of a tooth root.

Cephalometric image: A standardized, extraoral projection utilized in the scientific study of the measurements of the head.

Ceramic: Non-metal, non-resin inorganic refractory compounds processed at high temperatures (600°C/1112°F and above) and pressed, polished or milled—including porcelains, glasses, and glass-ceramics.

Chronic periradicular or chronic periapical abscess: An inflammatory reaction to pulpal infection and necrosis characterized by gradual onset, little or no discomfort and the intermittent discharge of pus through an associated sinus tract. May also be known as chronic alveolar abscess, chronic apical abscess, chronic dentoalveolar abscess, suppurative apical periodontitis, suppurative periradiucular periodontitis.

Cleft palate: Congenital deformity resulting in lack of fusion of the soft and/or hard palate, either partial or complete.

Clenching: The clamping and pressing of the jaws and teeth together in centric occlusion, frequently associated with psychological stress or physical effort.

Clinical crown: That portion of a tooth not covered by tissues.

Closed bite/Deep bite: Also known as deep overbite, this occurs when the upper front teeth overlap the bottom front teeth an excessive amount.

Closed reduction: The re-approximation of segments of a fractured bone without direct visualization of the bony segments.

Complete denture: A prosthetic for the edentulous maxillary or mandibular arch, replacing the full dentition. Usually includes six anterior teeth and eight posterior teeth.

Complete series: An entire set of radiographs. A set of intraoral radiographs usually consisting of 14 to 22 periapical and posterior bitewing images intended to display the crowns and roots of all teeth, periapical areas and alveolar bone crest (*Source*: FDA/ADA radiographic guidelines).

Composite: A dental restorative material made up of disparate or separate parts (e.g. resin and quartz particles).

Compound fracture: Break in bone which is exposed to external contamination.

Comprehensive treatment: Complete orthodontic treatment performed to correct a malocclusion.

Consultation: In a dental setting, a diagnostic service provided by a dentist where the dentist, patient, or other parties (e.g. another dentist, physician, or legal guardian) discuss the patient's dental needs and proposed treatment modalities.

Contiguous: Adjacent; touching.

Contract: A legally enforceable agreement between two or more individuals or entities that confers rights and duties on the parties. Common types of contracts include: 1) contracts between a dental benefit organization and an individual dentist to provide dental treatment to members of an alternative benefit plan. These contracts define the dentist's duties both to beneficiaries of the dental benefit plan and the dental benefit organization, and usually define the manner in which the dentist will be reimbursed; and 2) contracts between a dental benefit organization and a group plan sponsor. These contracts typically describe the benefits of the group plan and the rates to be charged for those benefits.

Contract dentist: Any dentist who has a contractual agreement with a dental benefit organization to render care to eligible persons.

Contract fee schedule plan: A dental benefit plan in which participating dentists agree to accept a list of specific fees for dental treatment provided.

Contract practice: A dental practice or organization that has a contractual arrangement with an insurer for the provision of services under an insurance contract.

Contract term: Usually, a 12 months period of time for which a contract is written and during which a group's deductibles, maximums and other provisions apply. This may or may not be the same as a calendar year. Also known as the benefit year.

Coping: A thin covering of the coronal portion of the tooth usually without anatomic conformity. Custom-made or pre-fabricated thimble-shaped core or base layer designed to fit over a natural tooth preparation, a post core, or implant abutment so as to act as a substructure onto which other components can be added to give final form to a restoration or prosthesis. It can be used as a definitive restoration or as part of a transfer procedure.

Core buildup: The replacement of a part or the entire crown of a tooth whose purpose is to provide a base for the retention of an indirectly fabricated crown.

Coronal: Refers to the crown of a tooth.

Cosmetic dentistry: Those services provided by dentists solely for the purpose of improving the appearance when form and function are satisfactory and no pathologic conditions exist [*Source*: ADA Policy Cosmetic Dentistry (1976:850)].

Cracked tooth syndrome: A collection of symptoms characterized by transient acute pain experienced when chewing.

Crossbite: Upper posterior (back) teeth are in crossbite, if they erupt and function inside or outside of the arch in the lower posterior teeth. Lower anterior (front) teeth are in crossbite, if they erupt and function in front of the upper anterior teeth. A crossbite can be individual teeth or groups of teeth.

Crown: An artificial replacement that restores missing tooth structure by surrounding the remaining coronal tooth structure, or is placed on a dental implant. It is made of metal, ceramic or polymer materials or a combination of such materials. It is retained by luting cement or mechanical means (*Source*: American College of Prosthodontics; The Glossary of Prosthodontic Terms).

Crown lengthening: A surgical procedure exposing more tooth for restorative purposes by apically positioning the gingival margin and removing supporting bone.

Culture and sensitivity test: Clinical laboratory test which identifies a microorganism and the ability of various antibiotics to control the microorganism.

Curettage: Scraping and cleaning the walls of a real or potential space, such as a gingival pocket or bone, to remove pathologic material.

Current dental terminology (CDT): The ADA reference manual that contains the Code on Dental Procedures and Nomenclature and other information pertinent to patient record-keeping and claim preparation by a dental office; published biennially (e.g. *CDT 2009–2010*).

Cusp: Pointed or rounded eminence on or near the masticating surface of a tooth.

Cuspid: Single-cusped tooth located between the incisors and bicuspids.

Cyst: Pathological cavity, usually lined with epithelium, containing fluid or soft matter.

Cytology: The study of cells including their anatomy, chemistry, physiology and pathology.

D

Debridement: Removal of subgingival and/or supragingival plaque and calculus which obstructs the ability to perform an evaluation; removal of contused and devitalized tissue from a wound surface.

Decay: The lay term for carious lesions in a tooth; decomposition of tooth structure.

Deciduous: Having the property of falling off or shedding; a term used to describe the primary teeth.

Deep sedation: A drug-induced depression of consciousness during which patients cannot be easily aroused but respond purposefully following repeated or painful stimulation. The ability to independently maintain ventilatory function may be impaired. Patients may require assistance in maintaining a patent airway, and spontaneous ventilation may be inadequate. Cardiovascular function is usually maintained.

Definitive prosthesis: Prosthesis to be used over an extended period of time.

Dental assessment: A limited clinical inspection that is performed to identify possible signs of oral or systemic disease, malformation, or injury, and the potential need for referral for diagnosis and treatment.

Dental home: The ongoing relationship between the dentist who is the Primary Dental Care Provider and the patient, which includes comprehensive oral health care, beginning no later than age one, pursuant to ADA policy.

Dental implant: A device especially designed to be placed surgically within or on the mandibular or maxillary bone as a means of providing for dental replacement.

Dental insurance: A plan that financially assists in the expense of treatment and care of dental disease and, in some cases, accidents to teeth.

Dental prepayment: A method of financing the cost of dental services prior to receiving the services.

Dental prosthesis: Any device or appliance replacing one or more missing teeth and/or, if required, associated structures (This is a broad term which includes abutment crowns and abutment inlays/onlays, bridges, dentures, obturators, gingival prostheses).

Dentin: Hard tissue which forms the bulk of the tooth and develops from the dental papilla and dental pulp, and in the mature state is mineralized.

Dentistry: The evaluation, diagnosis, prevention and/or treatment (nonsurgical, surgical or related procedures) of diseases, disorders and/or conditions of the oral cavity, maxillofacial area and/or the adjacent and associated structures and their impact on the human body; provided by a dentist, within the scope of his/her education, training and experience, in accordance with the ethics of the profession and applicable law.

Dentition: The teeth in the dental arch.

Deciduous dentition: Refers to the deciduous or primary teeth in the dental arch.

Denture: An artificial substitute for some or all of the natural teeth and adjacent tissues.

Denture base: That part of a denture that makes contact with soft tissue and retains the artificial teeth.

Diagnostic cast: Plaster or stone model of teeth and adjoining tissues; also referred to as study model. Primarily for use in extraoral examinations of relationships existing between oral tissues so as to determine how those relationships will effect form and function of a dental restoration or appliance being planned, or so as to determine whether subsequent predefinitive impression tissue treatment or modification might be necessary in order to insure optimal performance of the planned restoration or appliance.

Diagnosis-related groups (DRGs): A system of classifying hospital patients on the basis of diagnosis, consisting of distinct groupings. A DRG assignment to a case is based on the patient's: (1) Principal diagnosis; (2) Treatment procedures performed; (3) Age; (4) Gender; and (5) Discharge status.

Diagnostic records: The material and information that the orthodontist needs to properly diagnose and plan a patient's treatment. Diagnostic records may include a thorough patient health history, a visual examination of the teeth and supporting structures, plaster models of the teeth, a wax bite registration, extraoral and intraoral photographs, a panoramic and a cephalometric radiograph.

Diagnostic imaging: A visual display of structural or functional patterns for the purpose of diagnostic evaluation. May be photographic or radiographic.

Diastema: A space, such as one between two adjacent teeth in the same dental arch.

Direct pulp cap: Procedure in which the exposed vital pulp is treated with a therapeutic material, followed with a base and restoration, to promote healing and maintain pulp vitality.

Direct restoration: A restoration fabricated inside the mouth.

Discectomy: Excision of the intra-articular disc of a joint.

Displaced tooth: A partial evulsion of a tooth; may be mesial, distal, facial, lingual or incisal.

Distal: Surface or position of a tooth most distant from the median line of the arch.

Dressing: Medication, bandages or other therapeutic material applied to a wound.

Dry socket: Localized inflammation of the tooth socket following extraction due to infection or loss of blood clot; osteitis.

E

Early and Periodic Screening, Diagnosis and Treatment Program (EPSDT): A federal program that provides comprehensive health care for children through periodic screenings, diagnostic and treatment services.

Ecchymosis: A large splotchy hemorrhage under a surface that is greater than 1.0 cm. in diameter.

Ectopic eruption: Term used to describe a tooth or teeth that erupt in an abnormal position.

Edentulous: Without teeth.

Eligibility date: The date an individual and/or dependents become eligible for benefits under a dental benefit contract. Often referred to as effective date.

Enamel: Hard calcified tissue covering dentin of the crown of tooth.

Endodontics: Endodontics is the branch of dentistry which is concerned with the morphology, physiology and pathology of the human dental pulp and periradicular tissues. Its study and practice encompass the basic and clinical sciences including biology of the normal pulp, the etiology, diagnosis, prevention and treatment of diseases and injuries of the pulp and associated periradicular conditions.

Endodontist: A dental specialist who limits his/her practice to treating disease and injuries of the pulp and associated periradicular conditions.

Endosteal (Endosseous): Device placed into the alveolar and basal bone of the mandible or maxilla and transecting only one cortical plate.

Enteral: Any technique of administration in which the agent is absorbed through the gastrointestinal (GI) tract or oral mucosa (i.e. oral, rectal, sublingual).

Eposteal (Subperiosteal): Subperiosteal implant that conforms to the superior surface of an edentulous area of alveolar bone.

Equilibration: Reshaping of the occlusal surfaces of teeth to create harmonious contact relationships between the upper and lower teeth; also known as occlusal adjustment.

Erosions: Shallow surface defects that do not expose underlying connective tissue

Erythema: A scientific word for “redness” (eryth = red)

Erythematous lesions: A lesion with redness; a red lesion.

Evaluation: The patient assessment that may include gathering of information through interview, observation, examination, and use of specific tests that allows a dentist to diagnose existing conditions. Please refer to specific oral evaluation code descriptors for more complete definitions.

Evidence-based dentistry: An approach to oral health care that requires the judicious integration of systematic assessments of clinically relevant scientific data relating to the patient's oral and medical condition and history, with the dentist's clinical expertise and the patient's treatment needs and preferences.

Evulsion: Separation of the tooth from its socket due to trauma.

Excision: Surgical removal of bone or tissue.

Exclusions: Dental services not covered under a dental benefit program.

Exfoliative: Refers to a thin layer of epidermis shed from the surface.

Exostosis: Overgrowth of bone.

Expiration date: In dentistry, the date on which the dental benefit contract expires; the date an individual ceases to be eligible for benefits.

Extraoral: Outside the oral cavity.

Extracoronal: Outside the crown of a tooth.

Extraction: The process or act of removing a tooth or tooth parts.

Exudate: A material usually resulting from inflammation or necrosis that contains fluid, cells, and/or other debris.

F

Facebow: A wire appliance used with a nightbrace, or headgear. Primarily used to move the upper first molars back, creating room for crowded or protrusive front teeth. The facebow has an internal wire bow and an external wire bow. The internal bow attaches to the buccal tube on the upper molar bands inside the mouth and the outer bow attaches to the breakaway safety strap of the nightbrace.

Facial: The surface of a tooth directed towards the cheeks or lips (i.e. the buccal and labial surfaces) and opposite the lingual surface.

Fascia: Related to a sheet or band of fibrous connective tissue enveloping, separating or binding together muscles, organs and other soft tissue structures of the body.

Fee: The monetary value ascribed to a procedure delivered by a dentist to a patient. There are various terms that include the word or concept of a fee that are defined as follows.

Fistula: A connection between two surfaces; in the oral cavity, a pathway conducting pus to the mucosal surface.

Fistulous track: Another name for a "fistula."

Fiberotomy: A surgical procedure designed to sever fibers of attachment around the tooth, usually performed to reduce the potential for relapse or post-orthodontic treatment tooth movement.

Filling: A lay term used for the restoring of lost tooth structure by using materials such as metal, alloy, plastic or porcelain.

Fixed partial denture: A prosthetic replacement of one or more missing teeth cemented or otherwise attached to the abutment teeth or implant replacements.

Fixed prosthesis: Non-removable dental prosthesis which is solidly attached to abutment teeth, roots or implants.

Fixed-removable prosthesis: Combined prosthesis, one or more parts of which are fixed, and the other(s) attached by devices which allow their detachment, removal and reinsertion by the dentist only.

Flossing: An important part of daily home dental care. Flossing removes plaque and food debris from between the teeth, brackets and wires. Flossing keeps teeth and gums clean and healthy during orthodontic treatment.

Foramen: Natural opening into or through bone.

Fracture: The breaking of a part, especially of a bony structure; breaking of a tooth.

Freedom of choice: The concept that a patient has the right to choose any licensed dentist to deliver his or her oral health care without any type of coercion.

Frenum: Muscle fibers covered by a mucous membrane that attaches the cheek, lips and or tongue to associated dental mucosa.

Frenectomy: The surgical removal or repositioning of the frenum, the lip and tongue attachment located between the upper and lower front teeth. A large frenum attachment can cause spacing between top-front teeth or cause the tongue to be tied.

Furcation: The anatomic area of a multirooted tooth where the roots diverge.

G

Genetic test: Laboratory technique used to determine, if a person has a genetic condition or disease or is likely to get the disease.

General anesthesia: A drug-induced loss of consciousness during which patients are not arousable, even by painful stimulation. The ability to independently maintain ventilatory function is often impaired. Patients often require assistance in maintaining a patent airway, and positive pressure ventilation may be required because of depressed spontaneous ventilation or drug-induced depression of neuromuscular function. Cardiovascular function may be impaired.

Gingiva: Soft tissues overlying the crowns of unerupted teeth and encircling the necks of those that have erupted.

Gingivectomy: The excision or removal of gingiva.

Gingivitis: Inflammation of gingival tissue without loss of connective tissue.

Gingivoplasty: Surgical procedure to reshape gingiva.

Glass ionomer: Polyelectrolyte cement in which the solid powder phase is a fluoride-containing aluminosilicate glass powder to be mixed with polymeric carboxylic acid. The cement can be used to restore teeth, fill pits and fissures, lute and line cavities. It is also known as glass polyalkenoate cement, ionic polymer cement and polyelectrolyte cement.

Gold foil: Thin pure gold leaf that is self adhering when condensed into a cavity. One of the oldest restorative techniques, it is compacted or condensed into a retentive cavity form.

Graft: A piece of tissue or alloplastic material placed in contact with tissue to repair a defect or supplement a deficiency.

Guided tissue regeneration (GTR): A surgical procedure that uses a barrier membrane placed under the gingival tissue and over the remaining bone support to enhance regeneration of new bone.

Gummy smile: Showing an excessive amount of gingival (gum) tissue above the front teeth when smiling.

H

Headgear: An appliance worn outside of the mouth to provide traction for growth modification and tooth movement.

Herbst appliance: This appliance is used to move the lower jaw forward. It can be fixed or removable. When it is fixed, it is cemented to teeth in one or both arches using stainless steel crowns. An expansion screw may be used simultaneously to widen the upper jaw.

Hemisection: Surgical separation of a multi-rooted tooth.

Histopathology: The study of disease processes at the cellular level.

Hyperplastic: Pertaining to an abnormal increase in the number of cells in an organ or a tissue with consequent enlargement.

I

Imaging, diagnostic: This would include, but is not limited to, CAT scans, MRIs, photographs, radiographs, etc.

Immediate denture: Prosthesis constructed for placement immediately after removal of remaining natural teeth.

Impacted tooth: A tooth that does not erupt into the mouth or only erupts partially is considered impacted.

Implant: Material inserted or grafted into tissue.

Implantation, tooth: Placement of an artificial or natural tooth into an alveolus.

Incisal: Pertaining to the biting edges of the incisor and cuspid teeth.

Incisal angle: One of the angles formed by the junction of the incisal and the mesial or distal surfaces of an anterior tooth; called the mesioincisal and distoincisal angle respectfully.

Incision and drainage: The procedure of incising a fluctuant mucosal lesion to allow for the release of fluid from the lesion.

Incisor: A tooth for cutting or gnawing; located in the front of the mouth in both jaws.

Indirect pulp cap: Procedure in which the nearly exposed pulp is covered with a protective dressing to protect the pulp from additional injury and to promote healing and repair via formation of secondary dentin.

Indirect restoration: A restoration fabricated outside the mouth.

Inhalation: A technique of administration in which a gaseous or volatile agent is introduced into the lungs and whose primary effect is due to absorption through the gas/blood interface.

Inlay: An intracoronal dental restoration, made outside the oral cavity to conform to the prepared cavity, which restores some of the occlusal surface of a tooth, but does not restore any cusp tips. It is retained by luting cement. (*Source*: American College of Prosthodontics; The Glossary of Prosthodontic Terms)

Interim prosthesis: A provisional prosthesis designed for use over a limited period of time, after which it is to be replaced by a more definitive restoration.

Interceptive treatment: Orthodontic treatment performed to intercept a developing problem. Usually performed on younger patients that have a mixture of primary (baby) teeth and permanent teeth.

Intentional reimplantation: The intentional removal, radicular repair and replacement of a tooth into its alveolus.

International Classification of Diseases (ICD): Diagnostic codes designed for the classification of morbidity and mortality information for statistical purposes; for the indexing of hospital records by disease and operations; and for data storage and retrieval.

Interproximal: Between the adjoining surfaces of adjacent teeth in the same arch.

Intracoronal: Referring to "within" the crown of a tooth.

Intraoral: Inside the mouth.

Interproximal reduction: Removal of a small amount of enamel from between the teeth to reduce their width. It is also known as reproximation, slenderizing, stripping, enamel reduction or selective reduction.

J

Jaw: A common name for either the maxilla or the mandible.

K

Keratin: A protein present in all cuticular structures of the body, such as hair, epidermis and horns.

Keratinized gingiva: The oral surface of the gingiva extending from the mucogingival junction to the gingival margin. In gingival health, the coronal portion of the sulcular epithelium may also be keratinized.

Keratotic lesion: A lesion caused by excessive keratin production.

L

Labial: Pertaining to or around the lip.

Laminate veneer: A thin covering of the facial surface of a tooth usually constructed of tooth-colored material used to restore discolored, damaged, mis-shapen or misaligned teeth.

Lesion: An injury or wound; area of diseased tissue.

Ligating modules: A small elastic O-ring, shaped like a donut, used to hold the archwire in the bracket.

Limitations: Restrictive conditions stated in a dental benefit contract, such as age, length of time covered, and waiting periods, which affect an individual's or group's coverage. The contract may also exclude certain benefits or services, or it may limit the extent or conditions under which certain services are provided.

Line angle: An angle formed by the junction of two planes; used to designate the junction of two surfaces of a tooth, or of two walls of a tooth cavity preparation.

Lingual: Pertaining to or around the tongue; surface of the tooth directed toward the tongue; opposite of facial.

Lip bumper: A wire appliance used to move the lower molars back and the lower front teeth forward, creating room for crowded front teeth. The lip bumper is an internal wire bow that attaches to the buccal tubes on the cheek side of the lower molar bands inside the mouth. The front portion of the bow has an acrylic pad or bumper that rests against the inside of the lower lip. The lower lip muscles apply pressure to the bumper creating a force that moves the molars back.

Lip incompetence: The inability to close the lips together at rest, usually due to protrusive front teeth or excessively long faces.

Locus: A site or location.

Local anesthesia: The elimination of sensation, especially pain, in one part of the body by the topical application or regional injection of a drug.

M

Macule: A flat discolored lesion that is not raised above the surface.

Maintenance, periodontal: Therapy for preserving the state of health of the periodontium.

Malar: Pertaining to the cheek bone.

Malignant: Having the properties of dysplasia, invasion, and metastasis.

Masses: A large submucosal lesion.

Malocclusion: The term used in orthodontics to describe teeth that do not fit together properly. From Latin, the term means "bad bite."

Mandible: The lower jaw.

Mandibular canal: The passage which transmits vessels and nerves through the jaw to branches that distributes them to the teeth.

Maryland bridge: Fixed partial denture featuring conservative retainers which are resin bonded to abutments.

Maxilla: The upper jaw.

McCall Festoons: Life preserver shaped enlargements of the marginal gingiva; occurs on canine and premolar region.

Medicaid: A federal assistance program established as Title XIX under the Social Security Act of 1965 which provides payment for medical care for certain low income individuals and families. The program is funded jointly by the state and federal governments and administered by states.

Medically necessary care: The reasonable and appropriate diagnosis, treatment, and follow-up care (including supplies, appliances and devices) as determined and prescribed by qualified, appropriate healthcare providers in treating any condition, illness, disease, injury, or birth developmental malformations. Care is medically necessary for the purpose of: controlling or eliminating infection, pain, and disease; and restoring facial configuration or function necessary for speech, swallowing or chewing.

Medicament: Substance or combination of substances intended to be pharmacologically active, especially prepared to be prescribed, dispensed or administered by authorized personnel to prevent or treat diseases in humans or animals.

Medicament, topical: Pharmacological substance especially prepared to be applied on tissues of the oral cavity.

Medicare: A federal insurance program enacted in 1965 as Title XVIII of the Social Security Act that provides certain inpatient hospital services and physician services for all persons age 65 and older and eligible disabled individuals. The program is administered by the Centers for Medicare and Medicaid Services (CMS), previously known as the Health Care Financing Administration (HCFA).

Mesial: Nearer the middle line of the body or the surface of a tooth nearer the center of the dental arch.

Microabrasion: Mechanical removal of a small amount of tooth structure to eliminate superficial enamel discoloration defects.

Microorganisms: A minute living organism, such as a bacterium, fungus, yeast, virus or rickettsia.

Minimal sedation: A minimally depressed level of consciousness, produced by a pharmacological method, that retains the patient's ability to independently and continuously maintain an airway and respond normally to tactile stimulation and verbal command. Although cognitive function and coordination may be modestly impaired, ventilatory and cardiovascular functions are unaffected.

Mixed dentition: The dental developmental stage in children (approximately ages 6–12) when they have a mix of primary (baby) and permanent teeth.

Mixed radiolucency-radiopacity: A radiographic lesion composed of a mixture of radiolucencies and radiopacities; indicates a mixture of soft and hard tissues.

Moderate sedation: A drug-induced depression of consciousness during which patients respond purposefully to verbal commands, either alone or accompanied by light tactile stimulation. No interventions are required to maintain a patent airway, and spontaneous ventilation is adequate. Cardiovascular function is usually maintained.

Molar: Teeth posterior to the premolars (bicuspids) on either side of the jaw; grinding teeth, having large crowns and broad chewing surfaces.

Mouthguard: A removable device used to protect the teeth and mouth from injury caused by sporting activities. The use of a mouthguard is especially important for orthodontic patients.

Mucous membrane: Lining of the oral cavity as well as other canals and cavities of the body; also called "mucosa."

N

Necessary treatment: A necessary dental procedure or service as determined by a dentist, to either establish or maintain a patient's oral health. Such determinations are based on the professional diagnostic judgment of the dentist, and the standards of care that prevail in the professional community.

Nightguard: A removable appliance worn at night to help an individual minimize the damage or wear while clenching or grinding teeth during sleep.

Non-autogenous: A graft from donor other than patient.

O

Obturate: With reference to endodontics, refers to the sealing of the canal(s) of tooth roots during root canal therapy procedure with an appropriately prescribed material such as gutta-percha in combination with a suitable luting agent.

Obturator: A disc or plate which closes an opening; a prosthesis that closes an opening in the palate.

Occlusal: Pertaining to the biting surfaces of the premolar and molar teeth or contacting surfaces of opposing teeth or opposing occlusion rims.

Occlusal radiograph: An intraoral radiograph made with the film, phosphorous plate, emulsion or digital sensor being held between the occluded teeth.

Occlusal surface: A surface of a posterior tooth or occlusion rim that is intended to make contact with an opposing occlusal surface.

Occlusion: Any contact between biting or chewing surfaces of maxillary (upper) and mandibular (lower) teeth.

Odontogenic: Refers to tooth-forming tissues.

Odontogenic cyst: Cyst derived from the epithelium of odontogenic tissue (developmental, primordial).

Odontoplasty: Adjustment of tooth length, size, and/or shape; includes removal of enamel projections.

Onlay: A dental restoration made outside the oral cavity that covers one or more cusp tips and adjoining occlusal surfaces, but not the entire external surface. It is retained by luting cement.

Open bite: A malocclusion in which teeth do not make contact with each other. With an anterior open bite, the front teeth do not touch when the back teeth are closed together. With a posterior open bite, the back teeth do not touch when the front teeth are closed together.

Open reduction: Re-approximation of fractured bony segments accomplished through cutting the adjacent soft tissues and bone to allow direct access.

Operculectomy: Removal of the operculum.

Operculum: The flap of tissue over an unerupted or partially erupted tooth.

Oral: Pertaining to the mouth.

Oral and maxillofacial pathologist: A dental specialist whose practice is concerned with recognition, diagnosis, investigation and management of diseases of the oral cavity, jaws, and adjacent structures.

Oral and maxillofacial pathology: Oral pathology is the specialty of dentistry and discipline of pathology that deals with the nature, identification, and management of diseases affecting the oral and maxillofacial regions. It is a science that investigates the causes, processes, and effects of these diseases. The practice of oral pathology includes research and diagnosis of diseases using clinical, radiographic, microscopic, biochemical, or other examinations.

Oral and maxillofacial radiologist: A dental specialist whose practice is concerned with the production and interpretation of images and data produced by all modalities of radiant energy used for the diagnosis and management of diseases, disorders and conditions of the oral and maxillofacial region.

Oral and maxillofacial radiology: Oral and maxillofacial radiology is the specialty of dentistry and discipline of radiology concerned with the production and interpretation of images and data produced by all modalities of radiant energy that are used for the diagnosis and management of diseases, disorders and conditions of the oral and maxillofacial region.

Oral and maxillofacial surgeon: A dental specialist whose practice is limited to the diagnosis, surgical and adjunctive treatment of diseases, injuries, deformities, defects and esthetic aspects of the oral and maxillofacial regions.

Oral and maxillofacial surgery: Oral and maxillofacial surgery is the specialty of dentistry which includes the diagnosis, surgical and adjunctive treatment of diseases, injuries and defects involving both the functional and esthetic aspects of the hard and soft tissues of the oral and maxillofacial region.

Oral diagnosis: The determination by a dentist of the oral health condition of an individual patient achieved through the evaluation of data gathered by means of history taking, direct examination, patient conference, and such clinical aids and tests as may be necessary in the judgment of the dentist.

Oral health literacy: The degree to which individuals have the capacity to obtain, process and understand basic health information and services needed to make appropriate oral health decisions.

Orthodontist: A dental specialist whose practice is limited to the interception and treatment of malocclusion and other neuromuscular and skeletal abnormalities of the teeth and their surrounding structures.

Orthodontics and dentofacial orthopedics: Orthodontics and dentofacial orthopedics is the dental specialty that includes the diagnosis, prevention, interception, and correction of malocclusion, as well as neuromuscular and skeletal abnormalities of the developing or mature orofacial structures.

Orthognathic: Functional relationship of maxilla and mandible.

Orthodontic device: Apparatus used to support, align, prevent or correct deformities, or to improve the function of movable parts of the body.

Orthodontic retainer: Appliance to stabilize teeth following orthodontic treatment.

OSHA: Abbreviation for Occupational Safety and Health Administration. Federal Agency in the US responsible for making and enforcing employee safety regulations.

Osteoplasty: Surgical procedure that modifies the configuration of bone.

Osteotomy: Surgical cutting of bone.

Overdenture: A removable prosthetic device that overlies and may be supported by retained tooth roots or implants.

P

Palate: The hard and soft tissues forming the roof of the mouth that separates the oral and nasal cavities.

Palatal expander: A fixed or removable device used to make the upper jaw wider.

Palliative: Action that relieves pain but is not curative.

Panoramic radiograph: An extraoral projection whereby the entire mandible, maxilla, teeth and other nearby structures are portrayed on a single image, as if the jaws were flattened out.

Papilla: A small, thick, solid raised surface lesions; a thick papule.

Papoose board: A behavior management technique utilizing immobilization to control the actions of a patient who is receiving dental treatment.

Papule: A small, firm, raised surface lesion.

Parafunctional: Other than normal function or use.

Parenteral: A technique of administration in which the drug bypasses the gastrointestinal (GI) tract (i.e. intramuscular [IM], intravenous [IV], intranasal [IN], submucosal [SM], subcutaneous [SC], intraosseous [IO].)

Parulis: A raised suppurating mucosal lesion through which a fistula ends.

Patch: A flat discolored lesion that is not raised above the surface; same as a macule.

Partial denture: Usually refers to a prosthetic device that replaces missing teeth. See fixed partial denture or removable partial denture.

Patient: An individual who has established a professional relationship with a dentist for the delivery of dental health care. For matters relating to communication of information and consent, this term includes the patient's parent, caretaker, guardian, or other individual as appropriate under state law and the circumstances of the case.

Pediatric dentist: A dental specialist whose practice is limited to treatment of children from birth through adolescence, providing primary and comprehensive preventive and therapeutic oral health care; formerly known as a pedodontist.

Pediatric dentistry: Pediatric dentistry is an age-defined specialty that provides both primary and comprehensive preventive and therapeutic oral health care for infants and children through adolescence, including those with special healthcare needs.

Peer review: An evaluation of the quality and conduct of an individual's work by the individual's professional equals (peers) in order to resolve questions or disputes regarding the quality, or conduct of the work. Peer review, when applied to dentistry, is a process, consistently structured and implemented by organized dentistry, in which a dentist's professional equals (peers) resolve questions or disputes (regarding the quality or appropriateness of care provided by the dentist or the fairness of the fee the dentist charged in an individual case) by retrospectively evaluating the quality or appropriateness of care in relation to professional norms or criteria or evaluating the fee charged in relation to the dentist's fee for the given complexity and level of care provided.

Percentile: The number in a frequency distribution below which a certain percentage of fees will fall. For example, the 90th percentile is the number that divides the distribution of fees into the lower 90% and the upper 10%, or that fee level at which 90% of dentists charge that amount or less, and 10% more.

Periapical: The area surrounding the end of the tooth root.

Periapical cyst: An apical inflammatory cyst containing a sac-like epithelium-lined cavity that is open to and continuous with the root canal.

Periapical radiograph: A radiograph made by the intraoral placement of film, phosphorous plate, emulsion or digital sensor, for disclosing the apices of the teeth.

Pericoronal: Around the crown of a tooth.

Periodontal: Pertaining to the supporting and surrounding tissues of the teeth.

Periodontal disease: Inflammatory process of the gingival tissues and/or periodontal membrane of the teeth, resulting in an abnormally deep gingival sulcus, possibly producing periodontal pockets and loss of supporting alveolar bone.

Periodontal pocket: Pathologically deepened gingival sulcus; a feature of periodontal disease.

Periodontics: Periodontics is that specialty of dentistry which encompasses the prevention, diagnosis and treatment of diseases of the supporting and surrounding tissues of the teeth or their substitutes and the maintenance of the health, function and esthetics of these structures and tissues.

Periodontist: A dental specialist whose practice is limited to the treatment of diseases of the supporting and surrounding tissues of the teeth.

Periodontitis: Inflammation and loss of the connective tissue of the supporting or surrounding structure of teeth with loss of attachment.

Periodontium: Tissue complex comprising gingival, cementum, periodontal ligament, and alveolar bone which attaches nourishes and supports the tooth.

Periradicular: Surrounding a portion of the root of the tooth.

Permanent dentition (Adult dentition): Refers to the permanent teeth in the dental arch.

Permanent dentition: Refers to the permanent or adult teeth in the dental arch.

Petechiae: Small pin-point hemorrhages on a body surface.

Pin: A small metal rod, cemented or driven into dentin to aid in retention of a restoration.

Plaque: A soft sticky substance that accumulates on teeth composed largely of bacteria and bacterial derivatives. A thick flat-discolored lesion not raised above the surface; a thick macule.

Polyp: A smooth dome-shaped benign neoplasm of covering and lining epithelium.

Pontic: The term used for an artificial tooth on a fixed partial denture (bridge).

Prorcelain/ceramic: Refers to those non-metal, non-resin inorganic refractory compounds processed at high temperatures (600ºC/1112ºF and above) and pressed, polished or milled, including porcelains, glasses, and glass-ceramics.

Post: Rod-like component designed to be inserted into a prepared root canal space so as to provide structural support. This device can either be in the form of an alloy, carbon fiber or fiberglass, and posts are usually secured with appropriate luting agents.

Posterior: Refers to teeth and tissues towards the back of the mouth (distal to the canines); maxillary and mandibular premolars and molars. The designation of permanent posterior teeth in the Universal/National tooth numbering system include teeth 1 through 5 and 12 through 16 (maxillary), and 17 through 21 and 28 through 32 (mandibular); primary teeth in the Universal tooth numbering system are designated A, B, I and J (maxillary), and K, L, S and T (mandibular).

Precision attachment: Interlocking device, having a male component integrated into a removable prosthesis that fits precisely into a female component embedded in the body of abutment teeth or implant abutments, to stabilize or retain the prosthesis when it is seated in the mouth.

Predetermination: A process where a dentist submits a treatment plan to the payer before treatment begins. The payer reviews the treatment plan and notifies the dentist and patient of one or more of the following: patient's eligibility, covered services, amounts payable, co-payment and deductibles and plan maximums.

Premedication: The use of medications prior to dental procedures.

Preventive dentistry: Aspects of dentistry concerned with promoting good oral health and function by preventing or reducing the onset and/or development of oral diseases or deformities and the occurrence of orofacial injuries.

Prophylaxis: Removal of plaque, calculus and stains from the tooth structures. It is intended to control local irritational factors.

Prosthesis: Artificial replacement of any part of the body.

Prosthodontics: Prosthodontics is the dental specialty pertaining to the diagnosis, treatment planning, rehabilitation and maintenance of the oral function, comfort, appearance and health of patients with clinical conditions associated with missing or deficient teeth and/or oral and maxillofacial tissues using biocompatible substitutes.

Prosthodontist: A dental specialist whose practice is limited to the restoration of the natural teeth and/or the replacement of missing teeth with artificial substitutes.

Prosthodontic retainer: A part of a prosthesis that attaches a restoration to the abutment tooth, implant abutment, or implant.

Provisional: Formed or preformed for temporary purposes or used over a limited period; a temporary or interim solution; usually refers to a prosthesis or individual tooth restoration.

Public health dentist: A dentist whose practice is limited to the science and art of preventing and controlling dental diseases and promoting dental health through organized community efforts.

Public health dentistry: Dental public health is the science and art of preventing and controlling dental diseases and promoting dental health through organized community efforts. It is that form of dental practice which serves the community as a patient rather than the individual. It is concerned with the dental health education of the public, with applied dental research, and with the administration of group dental care programs as well as the prevention and control of dental diseases on a community basis.

Pulp: Connective tissue that contains blood vessels and nerve tissue which occupies the pulp cavity of a tooth.

Pulp cavity: The space within a tooth which contains the pulp.

Pulpectomy: Complete removal of vital and non-vital pulp tissue from the root canal space.

Pulpitis: Inflammation of the dental pulp.

Pulpotomy: Removal of a portion of the pulp, including the diseased aspect, with the intent of maintaining the vitality of the remaining pulpal tissue by means of a therapeutic dressing.

Purpura: Hemorrhage under a surface that is about 1.0 cm in diameter.

Q

Quadrant: One of the four equal sections into which the dental arches can be divided; begins at the midline of the arch and extends distally to the last tooth.

R

Radicular: Pertaining to the root.

Radiographic/surgical implant index: An appliance, designed to relate osteotomy or fixture position to existing anatomic structures.

Radiograph: An image or picture produced on a radiation sensitive film, phosphorous plate, emulsion or digital sensor by exposure to ionizing radiation.

Radiolucency: A dark area on a radiograph indicating presence of a material that does not impede passage of X-rays.

Radiopacity: A light area on a radiograph indicating presence of a material that impedes passage of X-rays.

Rebase: Process of refitting a denture by replacing the base material.

Recalcification: Procedure used to encourage biologic root repair of external and internal resorption defects.

Reimplantation, tooth: The return of a tooth to its alveolus.

Reline: Process of resurfacing the tissue side of a removable prosthesis with new base material.

Removable orthodontic appliance: An orthodontic appliance that can be removed from the mouth by the patient. Removable appliances are used to move teeth, align jaws and to keep teeth in their new positions when the braces are removed (retainers).

Removable partial denture: A removable partial denture is a prosthetic replacement of one or more missing teeth that can be removed by the patient.

Removable prosthesis: Complete or partial prosthesis, which after an initial fitting by a dentist, can be removed and reinserted by the patient.

Resin, acrylic: Resinous material of the various esters of acrylic acid, used as a denture base material, for trays or for other restorations.

Resin infiltration: Application of a resin material engineered to penetrate and fill the sub-surface pore system of an incipient caries lesion to strengthen, stabilize, and limit the lesion's progression, as well as mask visible white spots.

Retail store dentistry: Refers to dental services offered within a retail, department or drug store operation. Typically, space is leased from the store by a separate administrative group that, in turn, subleases to a dentist or dental group providing the actual dental services. The dental operation generally maintains the same hours of operation as the store and appointments often are not necessary. Considered to be a type of practice, not a dental benefit plan model.

Retrograde filling: A method of sealing the root canal by preparing and filling it from the root apex.

Retrospective review: A post-treatment assessment of services on a case-by-case or aggregate basis after the services have been performed.

Revision: The act of revising; second or more surgical procedure for correction of a condition.

Root: The anatomic portion of the tooth that is covered by cementum and is located in the alveolus (socket) where it is attached by the periodontal apparatus; radicular portion of tooth.

Residual root: Remaining root structure following the loss of the major portion (over 75%) of the crown.

Root canal: The portion of the pulp cavity inside the root of a tooth; the chamber within the root of the tooth that contains the pulp.

Root canal therapy: The treatment of disease and injuries of the pulp and associated periradicular conditions.

Root planing: A definitive treatment procedure designed to remove cementum and/or dentin that is rough, may be permeated by calculus, or contaminated with toxins or microorganisms.

Rubber bands: During certain stages of treatment, small elastics or rubber bands are worn to provide individual tooth movement or jaw alignment.

Rubber dam: A barrier technique used to prevent the passage of saliva or moisture, or to provide an isolated operative field.

S

Salivary gland: Exocrine glands that produce saliva and empty it into the mouth; these include the parotid glands, the submandibular glands and the sublingual glands.

Scaling: Removal of plaque, calculus, and stain from teeth.

Sealant: A resinous material designed to be applied to the occlusal surfaces of posterior teeth to prevent occlusal caries.

Sedative filling: A temporary restoration intended to relieve pain.

Semi-precision attachment: A device, one component of which is fixed to an abutment or abutments and the other is integrated into a fixed or removable prosthesis in order to stabilize and/or retain it.

Safety strap: The safety strap prevents the facebow of the headgear from coming loose and causing injury.

Separators: An elastic O-ring or small wire loop placed between the teeth to create space for placement of bands. Separators are usually placed between the teeth a week before bands are scheduled to be cemented to the teeth.

Serial extraction: Selective or guided removal of certain primary (baby) teeth and/or permanent teeth over a period of time to create room for permanent teeth.

Service corporations: Dental benefit organizations established under not-for-profit state statutes for the purpose of providing healthcare coverage, e.g. Delta Dental Plans, Blue Cross and Blue Shield Plans.

Sextant: One of the six relatively equal sections into which a dental arch can be divided, e.g. tooth numbers 1-5; 6-11; 12-16; 17-21; 22-27; 28-32. Sometimes used for recording periodontal charting.

Sialodochoplasty: Surgical procedure for the repair of a defect and/or restoration of portion of a salivary gland duct.

Sialography: Inspection of the salivary ducts and glands by radiograph after the injection of a radiopaque medium.

Sialolithotomy: Surgical procedure by which a stone within a salivary gland or its duct is removed, either intraorally or extraorally.

Site: A term used to describe a single area, position, or locus. For periodontal procedures, an area of soft tissue recession on a single tooth or an osseous defect adjacent to a single tooth; also used to indicate soft tissue defects and/or osseous defects in edentulous tooth positions.

Space maintainer: A fixed appliance used to hold space for an unerupted permanent tooth after a primary (baby) tooth has been lost prematurely, due to accident or decay.

Splint: A device used to support, protect, or immobilize oral structures that have been loosened, replanted, fractured or traumatized. Also refers to devices used in the treatment of temporomandibular joint disorders.

Steroid prep: A steroid prep is a controlled increase of glucocorticoids given prior to the patients' dental appointment which is slowly reduced to a normal dosage level over a 2–3 day period following therapy.

Still man's clefts: V-shaped indentations extending from free gingiva up to varying depths towards attached gingiva; occurs on the facial surfaces.

Stomatitis: Inflammation of the membranes of the mouth.

Stop-loss: A general term referring to that category of coverage that provides insurance protection (reinsurance) to an employer for a self-funded plan.

Stress breaker: That part of a tooth-borne and/or tissue-borne prosthesis designed to relieve the abutment teeth and their supporting tissues from harmful stresses.

Study model: Plaster or stone model of teeth and adjoining tissues; also referred to as diagnostic cast.

Succedaneous tooth: A permanent tooth that replaces a primary (deciduous) tooth.

Supernumerary teeth: A genetic occurrence in which there are more teeth than the usual number. These teeth can be malformed or erupt in abnormally.

Suture: Stitch used to repair incision or wound.

T

Telangiectasia: A group of dilated small blood vessels seen under a surface.

Temporary removable denture: An interim prosthesis designed for use over limited period of time.

Temporomandibular joint (TMJ): The connecting hinge mechanism between the base of the skull (temporal bone) and the lower jaw (mandible).

Temporomandibular joint dysfunction (TMD or TMJD): Abnormal functioning of temporomandibular joint; also refers to symptoms arising in other areas secondary to the dysfunction.

Therapeutic: Of or pertaining to therapy or treatment; beneficial. Therapy has as its goal the elimination or control of a disease or other abnormal state.

Tissue conditioning: Material intended to be placed in contact with tissues, for a limited period, with the aim of assisting the return to a healthy condition.

Tomography: An X-ray technique that produces an image representing a detailed cross-section of tissue structures at a predetermined depth.

Tongue thrust: An individual's tongue pushes against the teeth when swallowing. Forces generated by the tongue can move the teeth and bone and may lead to an anterior or posterior open bite.

Tongue crib: A fixed appliance used to help a patient stop habits or undesirable tongue forces exerted on the teeth and bone that supports the teeth.

Tooth-bounded space: A space created by one or more missing teeth that has a tooth on each side.

Torus: A bony elevation or protuberance of bone.

Tracheotomy: A surgical procedure to create an opening in the trachea (windpipe) to aid in breathing.

Transdermal: A technique of administration in which the drug is administered by patch or iontophoresis through skin.

Transmucosal: A technique of administration in which the drug is administered across mucosa such as intranasal, sublingual or rectal.

Transitional: Relating to a passage or change from one position, state, phase or concept to another.

Transitional dentition: Refers to a mixed dentition; begins with the appearance of the permanent first molars and ends with the exfoliation of the deciduous teeth.

Transitional dentition: Refers to a mixed dentition; begins with the appearance of the permanent first molars and ends with the exfoliation of the deciduous teeth.

Transosteal (Transosseous): Device with threaded posts penetrating both the superior and inferior cortical bone plates of the mandibular symphysis and exiting through the permucosa. It may be intraoral or extraoral.

Transplantation: Surgical placement of biological material from one site to another.

Transplantation of tooth: Transfer of a tooth from one socket to another, either in the same or a different person.

Transeptal: Through or across a septum.

Treatment plan: The sequential guide for the patient's care as determined by the dentist's diagnosis and is used by the dentist for the restoration to and/or maintenance of optimal oral health.

Trismus: Restricted ability to open the mouth, usually due to inflammation or fibrosis of the muscles of mastication.

Tuberosity: A protuberance on a bone.

U

Unerupted: Tooth/teeth that have not penetrated into the oral cavity.

Unilateral: One-sided; pertaining to or affecting but one side.

Universal/National tooth numbering system: A system that assigns a unique number (from 1-32) to permanent teeth, and a unique letter (A-T) for primary teeth.

V

Varicosities: Permanently distended veins.

Verruca: A raised surface lesion with many small projections; a warty surface lesion.

Vertical bitewing: A dental image with a central projection on which the teeth can close, holding it in a vertical position for the radiographic examination of several upper and lower teeth simultaneously.

Vertical dimension: The vertical height of the face with the teeth in occlusion or acting as stops.

Vestibuloplasty: Any of a series of surgical procedures designed to increase relative alveolar ridge height.

Viral culture: A collection of specimen for the purpose of incubating a virus for identification.

W

Waiting period: The period between employment or enrollment in a dental program and the date when a covered person becomes eligible for a given benefit.

Wax pattern: A wax form that is the positive likeness of an object to be fabricated.

Worker's compensation: A benefit paid to an employee who suffers a work-related injury or illness.

Wax: Wax is placed on the brackets or archwires to prevent them from irritating the lips or cheeks.

Wires: Also known as archwires, they are held in the brackets using small elastic O-rings or stainless steelwire ligatures. Wires are used to move the teeth.

X

Xerostomia: Decreased salivary secretion that produces a dry and sometimes burning sensation of the oral mucosa and/or cervical caries.

Y

Yeast: A general term for a fungus occurring as a unicellular, nucleated organism that usually reproduces by budding. Some yeasts may reproduce by fission, many producing mycelia or pseudomycelia.

Z

Zygomatic bone: Quadrangular bone on either side of face that forms the cheek prominence.

Bibliography

Aberg JA, Kaplan JE, Libman H, et al. HIV Medicine Association of the Infectious Diseases Society of America. Primary care guidelines for the management of persons infected with human immunodeficiency virus: 2009 update by the HIV medicine Association of the Infectious Diseases Society of America. Clin Infect Dis 2009;49(5):651-81.

Adamson JW. The anemia of inflammation/malignancy: Mechanisms and management. Hematology Am Soc Hematol Educ Program 2008.pp.159-65.

ADA Council on Scientific Affairs. Office emergencies and emergency kits. J Am Dent Assoc 2002;133(3):364-5.

Akintoye SO, Greenberg MS. Recurrent aphthous stomatitis. Dent Clin North Am 2005;49(1):31-47.

American Diabetes Association. Standards of medical care in diabetes-2009. Diabetes Care 2009;32:S13-61.

Andrews NC. Forging a field: the golden age of iron biology. Blood 2008;112(2):219-30.

Ansell J, Hirsh J, Poller L, et al. The pharmacology and management of the vitamin K antagonists: the Seventh ACCP Conference on Antithrombotic and Thrombolytic Therapy. Chest 2004;126(Suppl 3):204S-33S.

Antonelli JR, Hottel TL. Oral manifestations of renal osteodystrophy: case report and review of the literature. Spec Care Dentist 2003;23(1):28-34.

Antoniades DZ, Markopoulos AK, Andreadis D, et al. Ulcerative uremic stomatitis associated with untreated chronic renal failure: report of a case and review of the literature. Oral Surg Oral Med Oral Pathol Oral Radiol Endod 2006;101(5):608-13.

Aragon CE, Burneo JG. Understanding the patient with epilepsy and seizures in the dental practice. J Can Dent Assoc 2007;73(1):71-6.

Atherton GJ, Mc Caul JA, Williams SA. Medical emergencies in general dental practice in Great Britain. Part 1: Their prevalence over a 10-year period. Br Dent J 1999;186(2):72-9.

Barker LR, Burton JR, Zieve PD (Eds). Principles of Ambulatory Medicine. 6th edn. Philadelphia, Lippincott Williams and Wilkins, 2003.

Basi DL, Schmiechen NJ. Bleeding and coagulation problems in the dental patient. Hereditary disease and medication-induced risks. Dent Clin North Am 1999;43(3):457-70.

Basker RM, Davenport JC. Prosthetic Treatment of the Edentulous Patient, 4th edn. Blackwell Munksgaard: Oxford, 2002.

Bates CJ, Flewitt A, Prentice AM, Lamb WH, Whitehead RG. Efficacy of a riboflavin supplement given at fortnightly intervals to pregnant and lactating women in rural Gambia. Hum Nutr Clin Nutr 1983;37(6):427-32.

Becker DE. Management of immediate allergic reactions. Dent Clin North Am 1995;39(3):577-86.

Beckman HB, Frankel RM. The effect of physician behavior on the collection of data. Ann Intern Med 1984;101:693-6.

Benz R, Schmidt R, Kelly K, Wolfson M. Epoetin alfa once every 2 weeks is effective for initiation of treatment of anemia of chronic kidney disease. Clin J Am Soc Nephrol 2007;2(2):215-21.

Bennett CR. Monheim's local anesthesia and pain control in dental practice, 7th edn. CBS Publishers and Distributors.

Bennett JD. Emergency drug therapy: drugs and routes of administration. Dent Clin North Am 1995;39(3):501-21.

Beutler E. Glucose-6-phosphate dehydrogenase deficiency: a historical perspective. Blood 2008;111(1):16-24.

Blinder D, Manor Y, Martinowitz U, et al. Dental extractions in patients maintained on oral anticoagulant therapy: comparison of INR value with occurrence of postoperative bleeding. Int J Oral Maxillofac Surg 2001;30(6):518-21.

Blinder D, Manor Y, Marinowitz U, et al. Dental extractions in patients maintained on continued oral anticoagulant: comparison of local hemostatic modalities. Oral Surg Oral Med Oral Pathol Oral Radiol Endod 1999;88(2):137-40.

Blount SG Jr. Cyanosis: pathophysiology and differential diagnosis. Prog Cardiovasc Dis 1971;13:595-605.

Borgna-Pignatti C. Modern treatment of thalassaemia intermedia. Br J Haematol 2007;138(3):291-304.

Bohmer T, Mowé M. The association between atrophic glossitis and protein-calorie malnutrition in old age. Age Ageing 2000;29(1):47-50.

Bouquot JE, Nikai H. Lesions of the oral cavity. In: Gnepp DR (Ed). Diagnostic Surgical Pathology of the Head and Neck. Philadelphia, Pa: Saunders; 2001;141.

Bussel JB, Cheng G, Saleh MN, et al. Eltrombopag for the treatment of chronic idiopathic thrombocytopenic purpura. N Engl J Med 2007;357(22):2237-47.

Busschots GV, Milzman BI. Dental patients with neurologic and psychiatric concerns. Dent Clin North Am 1999;43(3):471-83.

Byrd JA, Bruce AJ, Rogers RS III. Glossitis and other tongue disorders. Dermatol Clin 2003;21(1):123-34.

Camisa C, Allen CM, Bowen B, Oslen RG. Indirect immunofluorescence of oral lichen planus, J Oral Pathol Med 1986;15:218-20.

Chan ES, Thornhill M, Zakrzewska J. Interventions for treating oral lichen planus. Cochrane Database Syst Rev 2000;(2):CD001168.

Chuang SF, Sung JM, Kuo SC, et al. Oral and dental manifestations in diabetic and nondiabetic uremic patient receiving hemodialysis. Oral Surg Oral Med Oral Pathol Oral Radiol Endod 2005;99(6):689-95.

Clinical manual for management of the HIV-infected adult. National AIDS Education and Training Centers National Resource Center. *http://www.aidsetc.org/aetc?page=cm-00-00*. Accessed November 30, 2009.

Clark MM, Album MM, Lloyd RW. Medical care of the dental patient. Am Fam Physician 1995;52(4):1126-32.

Clinician's Guide to HIV-infected Patients, 3rd edn. Patton LL (Ed). The American Academy of Oral Medicine, 2001.

Coleman GC. Principles of Oral Diagnosis. Mosby-Year Book: St. Louis, 1993.

Cooke BE. History of oral medicine. Br Dent J 1981;151(1):11-3.

Cooke BE. Median rhomboid glossitis: candidiasis and not a developmental anomaly. Br J Dermatol 1975;93(4):399-405.

Crispian S. Oral and Maxillofacial Medicine: The Basis of Diagnosis and Treatment. Wright: New York, 2004.

Daneshpazhooh M, Moslehi H, Akhyani M, Etesami M. Tongue lesions in psoriasis: a controlled study. BMC Dermatol 2004;4(1):16.

Daniel TE, White QC. Direct immunofluorescence in oral mucosal disease: a diagnostic analysis of 130 cases. Oral Surgery 1981;51:38-46.

Daniel JG. Advanced endodontics for clinicians. J & J Publishers.1998.pp.16-23

Delaunay J. The molecular basis of hereditary red cell membrane disorders. Blood Rev 2007;21(1):1-20.

De Rossi SS, Glick M. Dental considerations for the patient with renal disease receiving hemodialysis. J Am Dent Assoc 1996;127(2);211-9.

David FM, Miles SS, Thomas BF. Oral Diagnosis, Oral Medicine, 3rd edn. Lea and Febiger: Philadelphia, 1987.

Doberneck RC. The diagnostic yield of lymph node biopsy. Arch Surg 1983;118:1203-5.

Donald AK, Major MA Jr, Dean MH. Oral Diagnosis, 6th edn. Mosby: St. Louis, 1983.

Donald A Kerr, Major M Ash, H. Dean Millard: oral diagnosis. CV Mosby company, 6th edn. 1983.pp.280-309.

Douglas LR, Douglass JB, Sieck JO, et al. Oral management of the patient with end-stage liver disease and the liver transplant patient. Oral Surg Oral Med Oral Pathol Oral Radiol Endod 1998;86(1):55-64.

Drage LA, Rogers RS III. Burning mouth syndrome. Dermatol Clin 2003;21(1):135-45.

Drinnan AJ. Medical conditions of importance in dental practice. Int Dent J 1990;40(4):206-10.

Edgar WM, Mullane DMO. Saliva and oral health, 2nd edn. 1996.

Edmondson HD, Frame JW, Malins AF. Medical emergencies in dental practice: an update on drugs and the management of acute airway obstruction. Dent 1989;16(6):254-56.

Edmondson HD, Frame JW. Medical emergencies in general practice, 2nd edn. Cardiopulmonary emergencies. Dent 1986;13(6):263-8.

Edward VZ, Kutscher AH, Geroge AH. Diagnosis of Diseases of the Mouth and Jaws, 2nd edn. Lea and Febiger: Philadelphia, 1978.

Emery RW, Guttenberg SA. Management priorities and treatment strategies for medical emergencies in the dental office. Dent Clin North Am 1999;43(3):401-19.

Expert Committee on Biological Standardization. Requirements for thromboplastins and plasma used to control oral anticoagulant therapy. World Health Organ Tech Rep Ser 1983;33:81-105.

Farmer A, Wade A, Goyder E, et al. Impact of self monitoring of blood glucose in the management of patients with non-insulin treated diabetes: open parallel group randomized study. BMJ 2007;335(7611):132.

Ferguson DB. Current diagnostic uses of saliva. J Dent Res 1987;66:420-4.

Feldstein AC, Smith DH, Perrin N, et al. Reducing warfarin medication interactions: an interrupted time series evaluation. Arch Intern Med 2006;166(9):1009-15.

Firriolo FJ. Diabetes mellitus. In: Hupp JR, Williams TP, Firriolo FJ (Eds). Dental Clinical Advisor, 1st edn. St Louis, MO: Mosby; 2006.pp.72-5.

Fischbach FT, Dunning MB. A Manual of Laboratory and Diagnostic Tests. 8th edn. Philadelphia, PA: Lippincott, Williams and Wilkins. 2009;275:369-75.

Fischer DS, Singer DH, Feldman SM. Clubbing: a review, with emphasis on hereditary acropachy. Medicine 1964;43:459-77.

Firriolo FJ. Drug use in hepatic dysfunction. In: Hupp JR, Williams TP, Firriolo FJ (Eds). Dental Clinical Advisor, 1st edn. St Louis, MO: Mosby; 2006;476.

Finazzi G, Barbui T. How I treat patients with polycythemia vera? Blood 2007;109(12): 5104-11.

Firriolo FJ. Common helpful information for medical disease and conditions. In: Hupp JR, Williams TP, Firriolo FJ (Eds). Dental Clinical Advisor, 1st edn. St Louis, MO: Mosby; 2006;487.

Foitzik C, Daublander M, Vietor K, et al. Management and care of patients at risk in a surgical dental practice. Anesth Prog 1996;43(3):73-7.

Franklin S Wein. Endodontic therapy. Mosby company, 5th edn. 1996.pp.65-71

Freeman NS, King RA, Plezia RA, et al. Office emergencies: an outline of causes, symptoms, and treatment. J Am Dent Assoc 1977;94(1):91-6.

Fogarty PF, Stetler-Stevenson M, Pereira A, Dunbar CE. Large granular lymphocytic proliferation-associated cyclic thrombocytopenia. Am J Hematol 2005;79(4):334-6.

Gardner ES, Goldberg LH. Granular cell tumor treated with Mohs micrographic surgery: report of a case and review of the literature. Dermatol Surg 2001;27(8):772-4.

George L. Treatment of Oral Diseases: a Concise Textbook. Thieme: New York, 2005.

Germing U, Strupp C, Kuendgen A, et al. Prospective validation of the WHO proposals for the classification of myelodysplastic syndromes. Haematologica. 2006;91(12): 1596-604.

Gies WJ. Dental education in the United States and Canada: a report to the Carnegie Foundation for the Advancement of Teaching. Carnegie Foundation: New York, Bulletin 19. 1926.

Glick M. Medical considerations for dental care of patients with alcohol-related liver disease. J Am Dent Assoc 1997;128(1):61-70.

Glick M. Oral diseases of HIV-associated immune suppression (ODHIS): a new classification system. Journal of Japanese Society for Oral Mucous Membrane 2004;10(2):56.

Goss AN. The dental management of medically compromised patients. Int Dent J 1984;34(4):227-31.

Godkar P. Textbook of Medical laboratory technology, 2nd edn. 2003.pp.251-77.

Go AS, Chertow GM, Fan D, et al. Chronic kidney disease and the risks of death, cardiovascular events, and hospitalization. N Engl J Med 2004;351(13):1296-305.

Golla K, Epstein JB, Cabay RJ. Liver disease: current perspectives on medical and dental management. Oral Surg Oral Med Oral Pathol Oral Radiol Endod 2004;98(5):516-21.

Greer JP, Foerster J, Rodgers GM, et al. Wintrobe's Clinical Hematology, 12th edn. Philadelphia, PA: Lippincott, Williams and Wilkins; 2008.

Grines CL, Bonow RO, Casey DE Jr, et al. Prevention of premature discontinuation of dual antiplatelet therapy in patients with coronary artery stents: a science advisory from the American Heart Association, American College of Cardiology, Society for Cardiovascular Angiography and Interventions, American College of Surgeons, and American Dental Association, with representation from the American College of Physicians. Circulation 2007;115(6):813-8.

Grushka M, Epstein JB, Gorsky M. Burning mouth syndrome. Am Fam Physician 2002;65(4):615-20.

Glickman's Clinical Periodontology, 7th edn. Carranza FA (Ed). WB Saunders Co: Philadelphia, PA, 1990.

Greenberger NJ. Gastrointestinal disorders, 3rd edn. Chicago: Year Book Medical Publishers, 1986.

Grossman RI, Youssem DM. Neuroradiology: The Requisites. Mosby: St. Louis, MO, 1994.

Hashimoto K, Kawashima S, Araki M, et al. Comparison of image performance between cone-beam computed tomography for dental use and four-row multidetector helical CT. J Oral Sci 2006;48(1):27-34.

Gonsalves WC, Chi AC, Neville BW. Common oral lesions: Part I. Superficial mucosal lesions. Am Fam Physician 2007;75(4):501-7.

Greenwood M. Medical emergencies in the dental practice. Periodontol 2000 2008;46:27-41.

Greenberg MS, Glick M. Burket's Oral Medicine, diagnosis and Treatment, 10th edn. 2003.

Gupta A, Epstein JB, Cabay RJ. Bleeding disorders of importance in dental care and related patient management. J Can Dent Assoc 2007;73(1):77-83.

Halstead CL, Blozis GG, Drinnan AJ, Gier RE. Physical evaluation of dental patient. CV Mosby company. 1982.pp.372-6.

Hamblin TJ. Autoimmune complications of chronic lymphocytic leukemia. Semin Oncol 2006;33(2):230-9.

Harrison's Principles of Internal Medicine, 17th edn. New York: McGraw-Hill; 2008.

Harold JJ, David KM. Oral Manifestations of Systemic Disease, 2nd edn. Bailliere Tindal: London, 1990.

Haslett C, Chilvers ER, Hunter JAA, Boon NA. Davidson's principles and practice of medicine, 18th edn. 1999.

Headstrom PD, Rulyak SJ, Lee SD. Prevalence of and risk factors for vitamin B_{12} deficiency in patients with Crohn's disease. Inflamm Bowel Dis 2008;14(2):217-23.

Henry JB. Clinical diagnosis and management by laboratory methods, 1999.

Hershey SE, Bayleran ED. Problem-oriented orthodontic record. J Clin Orthod 1986;20:106–10.

Hirsh J, Guyatt G, Albers GW, et al. American College of Chest Physicians. Antithrombotic and thrombolytic therapy: American College of Chest Physicians Evidence-Based Clinical Practice Guidelines, 8th edn. Chest 2008;133(Suppl 6):110S-2S.

Hovinga J, Roodvoets AP, Gaillard J. Some findings in patients with uraemic stomatitis. J Maxillofac Surg 1975;3(2):125-7.

Hruska KA. Renal osteodystrophy. In: Goldman L, Ausiello D (Eds). Cecil's Textbook of Medicine, 23rd edn. Philadelphia, PA: WB Saunders; 2007.pp.931-6.

Hunder GG. Giant cell (temporal) arteritis. Rheum Dis Clin North Am 1990;16(2):399-409.

Hurst JW, Morris DC, Crawley IS. The history: symptoms due to cardiovascular disease. In: Hurst JW, Logue RB, Rackley CE, Schlant RC, Sonnenblick, EH, Wallace AC, Wenger NK (Eds). The heart. 6th edn. New York: McGraw-Hill. 1985;7.

Hutchison's Clinical Methods. Sir Robert Hutchison, Michael Swash (Eds). Bailliere Tindall, 1989.

Hunder GG. Giant cell (temporal) arteritis. Rheum Dis Clin North Am 1990;16(2):399-409.

Hvas AM, Nexo E. Diagnosis and treatment of vitamin B_{12} deficiency: an update. Haematologica 2006;91(11):1506-12.

Hamid MJ, Dummer CD, Pinto LS. Systemic conditions, oral findings and dental management of chronic renal failure patients: general considerations and case report. Braz Dent J 2006;17(2):166-70.

Irwin D, Mandel IE. Salivary diagnosis: more than a lick and a promise. J Am Dent Assoc 1993;124:85-7.

Jackson DL, Johnson BS. Conscious sedation for dentistry: risk management and patient selection. Dent Clin North Am 2002;46(4):767-80.

Jainkittivong A, Yeh CK, Guest GF, et al. Evaluation of medical consultations in a predoctoral dental clinic. Oral Surg Oral Med Oral Pathol Oral Radiol Endod 1995;80(4):409-13.

James R Fricton, Richard J Kroening, Kate M Hathaway. TMJ and craniofacial pain: diagnosis and management, 1st edn. Ishiyaku Euroamerica Inc. 1988.

Jenkin's Physiology and biochemistry, 4th edn. 318-24.

John V Dacie, SM Lewis. Practical haematology. Harcourt Brace and Company Ltd, 8th edn. 1999.

Joseph BK, Savage NW. Tongue pathology. Clin Dermatol 2000;18(5):613-8.

Jones AS, Rafferty M, Fenton JE, Jones TM, Husband DJ. Treatment of squamous cell carcinoma of the tongue base: irradiation, surgery, or palliation? Ann Otol Rhinol Laryngol 2007;116(2):92-9.

Jolly DE. Evaluation of the medical history. Dent Clin North Am 1994;38(3):361-80.

Jolly DE. Recognition of medical risk in the dental patient. Anesth Prog 1995;42 (3-4):90-2.

Jowett NI, Cabot LB. Patients with cardiac disease: considerations for the dental practitioner. Br Dent J 2000;189(6):297-302.

Jungell P, Malmstrom M, Wartiovvara J. Light, Electrons immunofluorescence microscope: features of OLP, lupus erythematous, leukoplakia proc. Finn Dent Soc 1984;80:107-4.

Kansal P, Sakati N, Rifai A, Woodhouse N. Lingual thyroid: diagnosis and treatment. Arch Intern Med 1987;147(11):2046-8.

Kasper DL, Braunwald E, Fauci AS, Hauser SL, Longo DL, Jameson JL, Loscalzo Hendler BH, Rose LF. Common medical emergencies: a dilemma in dental education. J Am Dent Assoc 1975;91(3):575-82.

Kasper DL, Harrison TR (Eds). Harrison's Principles of Internal Medicine, 16th edn. New York, McGraw-Hill, 2005.

Kauffman E, Lamster IB. The diagnostic applications of saliva: a review. Crit Rev Oral Boil Med 2002;13:197-212.

Kellett M. Oral white plaques in uraemic patients. Br Dent J 1983;154(11):366-8.

Kerr AR. Update on renal disease for the dental practitioner. Oral Surg Oral Med Oral Pathol Oral Radiol Endod 2001;92(1):9-16.

Killip S, Bennett JM, Chambers MD. Iron deficiency anemia. Am Fam Physician 2007;75(5):671-8.

Klastersky J, Paesmans M, Georgala A, et al. Outpatient oral antibiotics for febrile neutropenic cancer patients using a score predictive for complications. J Clin Oncol 2006;24(25):4129-34.

Kroenke K. The case presentation: stumbling blocks and stepping stones. Am J Med 1985;79(5):605-8.

Kuderer NM, Dale DC, Crawford J, Lyman GH. Impact of primary prophylaxis with granulocyte colony stimulating factor on febrile neutropenia and mortality in adult cancer patients receiving chemotherapy: a systematic review. J Clin Oncol 2007;25(21):3158-67.

Lamb E. Top 200 drugs of 2008. Pharmacy Times. 2009 (May), Published online at http:// *www.pharmacytimes.com/issue/pharmacy/2009/2009/RxFocusTop200Drugs-0509. Accessed January 20, 2010.*

Lamey PJ, Lamb AB. Prospective study of aetiological factors in burning mouth syndrome. Br Med J (Clin Res Ed) 1988;296(6631):1243-6.

Larheim TA. Role of magnetic resonance imaging in the clinical diagnosis of the temporomandibular joint. Cells Tissues Organs 2005;180(1):6-21.

Lavelle CR. Applied oral physiology. Butterworths and Co. Ltd, 2nd edn. 1988.pp.136-7.

Leitner JM, Graninger W, Thalhammer F. Hepatotoxicity of antibacterials: pathomechanisms and clinical data. Infection 2010;38(1):3-11.

Lee HJ, Jo DY. Images in clinical medicine. a smooth, shiny tongue. N Engl J Med 2009;360(6):e8.

Leão JC, Gueiros LA, Segundo AV, et al. Uremic stomatitis in chronic renal failure. Clinics (Sao Paulo) 2005;60(3):259-62.

Lee JJ, Hung HC, Cheng SJ, et al. Carcinoma and dysplasia in oral leukoplakias in Taiwan: prevalence and risk factors. Oral Surg Oral Med Oral Pathol Oral Radiol Endod 2006;101(4):472-80.

Lindeman RD, Tobin J, Shock NW. Longitudinal studies on the rate of decline in renal function with age. J Am Geriatr Soc 1985;33(4):278-85.

Little JW, Falace DA, Miller CS, et al. Dental management of the medically compromised patient, 7th edn. St Louis, MO: Mosby; 2008;147:190.

Llewellyn CD, Johnson NW, Warnakulasuriya KA. Risk factors for squamous cell carcinoma of the oral cavity in young people: a comprehensive literature review. Oral Oncol 2001;37(5):401-8.

Louis I Grossman, Saymour Oliet, Carlos E Delrio. Endodontic practice. Varghese Publishing House, 11th edn. 1988.pp.12-8.

Lync MA, Brightman VJ, Greenberg MS. Burket's Oral Medicine: diagnosis and Treatment, 8th edn, 1984.

Lync MA, Brightman VJ, Greenberg MS. Burket's Oral Medicine: diagnosis and Treatment, 9th edn, 1998.

Maiti CR. A concise note on medical laboratory technology, 1995.

Malamed SF. Back to basics: emergency medicine in dentistry. J Calif Dent Assoc 1997;25(4):285-6,288-94.

Malamed SF. Emergency medicine in pediatric dentistry: preparation and management. J Calif Dent Assoc 2003;31(10):749-55.

Malamed SF. Medical Emergencies in the Dental Office, 5th edn. St Louis: Mosby, 2000.

Mandel IP. The diagnostic uses of saliva. J Oral Pathol Med 1990;19:119-25.

Manji I. Managing emergency patients. J Can Dent Assoc 1995;61(8):662-3.

Mask AG Jr. Medical management of the patient with cardiovascular disease. Periodontol 2000;23:136-41.

Massry S, Smogorzewski M. Dysfunction of PMN leukocytes in uremia: role of PTH. Kidney Int 2001;Suppl 78:195-6.

McCrae KR. Thrombocytopenia in pregnancy. Hematology Am Soc Hematol Educ Program 2010;2010:397-402.

McDaniel TF, Miller D, Jones R, et al. Assessing patient willingness to reveal health history information. J Am Dent Assoc 1995;126:375.

McGrath EE, Bardsley P, Basran G. Black hairy tongue: what is your call? CMAJ 2008;178(9):1137-8.

Mehra P, Caiazzo A. Maloney P. Lidocaine toxicity. Anesth Prog 1998;45(1):38-41.

Michota FA, Frost SD. The preoperative evaluation: use the history and physical rather than routine testing. Cleve Clin J Med 2004;71(1):63-70.

Miller CS, McGarity GJ. Tetracycline-induced renal failure after dental treatment. J Am Dent Assoc 2009;140(1):56-60.

Miller HJ, Hu J, Valentine JK, Gable PS. Efficacy and tolerability of intravenous ferric gluconate in the treatment of iron deficiency anemia in patients without kidney disease. Arch Intern Med 2007;167(12):1327-8.

Mirowski GW, Mark LA. Oral disease and oral-cutaneous manifestations of gastrointestinal and liver disease. In: Feldman M, Friedman LS, Brandt LJ (Eds). Sleisenger and Fordtran's Gastrointestinal and Liver Disease, 8th edn. Philiadephia, Pa: Saunders; 2006.pp.443-59.

Mitch WE. Chronic kidney disease. In: Goldman L, Ausiello D (Eds). Cecil's Textbook of Medicine, 23rd edn. Philadelphia, PA: WB Saunders; 2007.pp.931-6.

Moore PA. Preventing local anesthesia toxicity. J Am Dent Assoc 1992;123(9):60-4.

Morrison AD, Goodday RH. Preparing for medical emergencies in the dental office. J Can Dent Assoc 1999;65(5):284-6.

Moskowitz L. Cardiac disease and hypertension: considerations for office treatment. Dent Clin North Am 1999;43(3):495-512.

Mooney MA, Janniger CK. Pyogenic granuloma. Cutis 1995;55(3):133-6.

Morimoto Y, Ono K, Tanaka T, et al. The functional evaluation of salivary glands using dynamic MR sialography following citric acid stimulation: a preliminary study. Oral Surg Oral Med Oral Pathol Oral Radiol Endod 2005;100(3):357-64.

Mosca NG, Rose Hathorn A. HIV-positive patients: dental management considerations. Dent Clin North Am 2006;50(4):635-57.

Moder KG. Use and interpretation of rheumatologic tests: a guide for clinicians. Mayo Clin Proc 1996;71(4):391-6.

Napier SS, Speight PM. Natural history of potentially malignant oral lesions and conditions: an overview of the literature. J Oral Pathol Med 2008;37(1):1-10.

National Kidney Foundation (NKF), KDOQI Clinical Practice Guidelines for Chronic Kidney Disease: Evaluation, Classification, and Stratification. Chronic Kidney Disease Guidelines. Part 4. Definition and classification of stages of chronic kidney disease. 2002. Available at: *www.kidney.org/professionals/KDOQI/guidelines_ckd/p4_class_g1.htm*. Accessed June 22, 2009.

Naylor GD, Fredericks MR. Pharmacologic considerations in the dental management of the patient with disorders of the renal system. Dent Clin North Am 1996;40(3):665-83.

Napeñas JJ, Hong CH, Brennan MT, et al. The frequency of bleeding complications after invasive dental treatment in patients receiving single and dual antiplatelet therapy. J Am Dent Assoc 2009;140(6):690-5.

New York Heart Association, Criteria Committee. Nomenclature and criteria for diagnosis of diseases of the heart and great vessels, 8th edn. Boston: Little, Brown, 1979.

Niwa H, Sato Y, Matsuura H. Safety of dental treatment in patients with previously diagnosed acute myocardial infarction or unstable angina pectoris. Oral Surg Oral Med Oral Pathol Oral Radiol Endod 2000;89(1):35-41.

O'Kane MJ, Bunting B, Copeland M, et al. ESMON study group. Efficacy of self monitoring of blood glucose in patients with newly diagnosed type 2 diabetes (ESMON study): randomised controlled trial. BMJ 2008;336(7654):1174-7.

Okeson JP. Bell's orofacial pains. Quintessence Publishing, 5th edn. 1995.pp.177-80.

Ozgursoy OB, Karatayli Ozgursoy S, Tulunay O, Kemal O, Akyol A, Dursun G. Melkersson-Rosenthal syndrome revisited as a misdiagnosed disease. Am J Otolaryngol 2009;30(1):33-7.

Patton LL, Shugars DA, Bonito AJ. A systematic review of complication risks for HIV-positive patients undergoing invasive dental procedures. J Am Dent Assoc 2002;133(2):195-201.

Pastore L, Carroccio A, Compilato D, Panzarella V, Serpico R, Lo Muzio L. Oral manifestations of celiac disease. J Clin Gastroenterol 2008;42(3):224-32.

Peter R. Sudden unconsciousness during local anesthesia. Anesth Pain Control Dent 1993;2(3):140-2.

Piecuch JF, Lieblich SE. Neurologic emergencies. Dent Clin North Am 1995;39(3):567-75.

Riley CK, Terezhalmy GT. The patient with hypertension. Quintessence Int 2001;32(9):671-90.

PJ Mehta's practical medicine for students and practitioners, 6th edn. 2003.pp.389-405.

Proctor R, Kumar N, Stein A, et al. Oral and dental aspects of chronic renal failure. J Dent Res 2005;84(3):199-205.

Raja K, Coletti DP. Management of the dental patient with renal disease. Dent Clin N Am 2006;50(4):529-45.

Rama Rao. AVSS. A textbook of biochemistry, 1990.

Ravikiran O, Praveen BN. Clinical Manual for Oral Medicine and Radiology, 1st edn. Jaypee Brothers Medical Publishers, India, 2007.

Refaat M, Hyle E, Malhotra R, Seidman D, Dey B. Linezolid-induced lingua villosa nigra. Am J Med 2008;121(6):e1.

Reiner A, Goldman HS. Oral medicine: a history and a point of view. NY State Dent J 1993;59(3):22-3.

RR Ananthanarayan, CKJ Paniker. Textbook of microbiology, 6th edn, 2000.

Rogers RS III, Bruce AJ. The tongue in clinical diagnosis. J Eur Acad Dermatol Venereol 2004;18(3):254-9.

Rodbard HW, Blonde L, Braithwaite SS, et al. AACE Diabetes Mellitus Practice Guidelines Task Force. American Association of Clinical Endocrinologists medical guidelines for clinical practice for the management of diabetes mellitus. Endocr Pract 2007;13(Suppl 1):S3-S68.

Ross WF 3rd, Salisbury PL 3rd. Uremic stomatitis associated with undiagnosed renal failure. Gen Dent 1994;42(5):410-2.

Ruggeri M, Rodeghiero F, Tosetta A, et al. Postsurgery outcomes in patients with polycythemia vera and essential thrombocythemia: a retrospective survey. Blood 2008;111(2):666-71.

Russell IJ, Hendricson WD, Harris GD, Gobert DV. A comparison of two methods for facilitating clinical data integration by medical students. Acad Med 1990;65(5):333-401.

Sakoda S, Kodama Y, Shiba R. Lymphoepithelial cyst of oral cavity: report of a case and review of the literature. Int J Oral Surg 1983;12(2):127-31.

Saef SH. Assessment of the medical emergency. Dent Clin North Am 1995;39(3):487-99.

Satya Narayana. A textbook of biochemistry, 2003.

Satish Gupte. Short textbook of medical microbiology, 7th edn, 1999.

Sam Frankel, Stanley Reitman, Alex C. Sonnwirth-Gradwohl's clinical laboratory methods and diagnosis, Volume 1, 7th edn, 1970.

Sarti GM, Haddy RI, Schaffer D, Kihm J. Black hairy tongue. Am Fam Physician 1990;41(6):1751-5.

Schiffrin EL, Lipman ML, Mann JF. Chronic kidney disease: effects on the cardiovascular system. Circulation 2007;116(1):85-97.

Schwartz RN. Anemia in patients with cancer: incidence, causes, impact, management, and use of treatment guidelines and protocols. Am J Health Syst Pharm 2007;64(3 Suppl 2):S5-S13.

Segal LM, Stephenson R, Dawes M, Feldman P. Prevalence, diagnosis, and treatment of ankyloglossia: methodologic review. Can Fam Physician 2007;53(6):1027-33.

Shafer DM. Respiratory emergencies in the dental office. Dent Clin North Am 1995;39(3):541-54.

Shah N. Taking a history: conclusion and closure. Student BMJ 2005;13:358-9.

Shampaine GS. Patient assessment and preventive measures for medical emergencies in the dental office. Dent Clin North Am 1999;43(3):383-400.

Sherin N, Simi T, Shameena P, Sudha S. Changing trends in oral cancer. Indian J Cancer 2008;45(3):93-6.

Shirlaw PJ, Chikte U, MacPhail L, et al. Oral and dental care and treatment protocols for the management of HIV-infected patients. Oral Dis 2002;8(Suppl 2):136-43.

Smith HW. Comparative physiology of the kidney. In: The Kidney: Structure and Function in Health and Disease. New York, NY: Oxford University Press, 1951. pp.520-74.

Solnitzsky OC, Jeghers H. Lymphadenopathy and disorders of the lymphatic system. In: MacBryde CM. Blacklow RS. Signs and symptoms: applied pathologic physiology and clinical interpretation, 5th edn. Philadelphia: JB Lippincott. 1970.pp.476-538.

Stern M, Buser AS, Lohri A, et al. Autoimmunity and malignancy in hematology: more than an association. Crit Rev Oncol Hematol 2007;63(2):100-10.

Stoya G, Gruhn B, Vogelsang H, et al. Flow cytometry as a diagnostic tool for hereditary spherocytosis. Acta Haematol 2006;116(3):186-91.

Streckfur CF, Bigler LR. Saliva as a diagnostic fluid. J Oral diseases. 2002;8:69-76.

Stephen Cohen, Richard C. Burns. Pathways of pulp. Mosby company, 8th edn. 2002. pp.12-26.

Shulman JD, Beach MM, Rivera-Hidalgo F. The prevalence of oral mucosal lesions in U.S. adults: data from the Third National Health and Nutrition Examination Survey, 1988-1994. J Am Dent Assoc 2004;135(9):1279-86.

Stride P, Scully P. Better ways of learning. Student BMJ 2005;13:360-1.

Taibah K, Ahmed M, Baessa E, Saleem M, Rifai A, al-Arifi A. An unusual cause of obstructive sleep apnoea presenting during pregnancy. J Laryngol Otol 1998;112(12):1189-91.

Tefferi A. Classification, diagnosis and management of myeloproliferative disorders in the JAK2V617F era. Hematology Am Soc Hematol Educ Program 2006.pp.240-5.

Terai H, Shimahara M. Atrophic tongue associated with *Candida*. J Oral Pathol Med 2005;34(7):397-400.

The Diagnosis, Evaluation and Management of von Willebrand Disease. Bethesda, MD: National Heart, Lung, and Blood Institute; December 2007. NIH Pub. No. *08-5832. www.nhlbi.nih.gov/guidelines/vwd/vwd.pdf.*

The Monograph Series on Oral Treatment of HIV+ Patients in Private Practice. Denver, Colorado: Howard Dental Center for HIV/AIDS Oral Medicine; 2006.

Thomson PD, Melmon KL, Richardson JA, et al. Lidocaine pharmacokinetics in advanced heart failure, liver disease, and renal failure in humans. Ann Intern Med 1973;78(4):499-508.

Thomason R. Treating asthmatic patients: the facts. J Calif Dent Assoc 2007;35(5):320-2.

van der Waal I, Schepman KP, van der Meij EH, Smeele LE. Oral leukoplakia: a clinicopathological review. Oral Oncol 1997;33(5):291-301.

van Diermen DE, Aartman IH, Baart JA, et al. Dental management of patients using antithrombotic drugs: critical appraisal of existing guidelines. Oral Surg Oral Med Oral Pathol Oral Radiol Endod 2009;107(5):616-24.

Venkatraman BK. Guest editorial in JIAOMR 2003;15(3).

Vernillo AT. Diabetes mellitus: relevance to dental treatment. Oral Surg Oral Med Oral Pathol Oral Radiol Endod 2001;91(3):263-70.

Vernillo AT. Dental considerations for the treatment of patients with diabetes mellitus. J Am Dent Assoc 2003;134:24S-33S.

Vesterinen M, Ruokonen H, Leivo T, et al. Oral health and dental treatment of patients with renal disease. Quintessence Int 2007;38(3):211-9.

Wahl MJ. Dental surgery in anticoagulated patients. Arch Intern Med 1998;158(15):1610-6.

Walker HK, Hall WD, Hurst JW, (Eds). Clinical Methods: The History, Physical, and Laboratory Examinations. 3rd en. Boston: Butterworths; 1990.

Ward KA, Napier SS, Winter PC, Maw RD, Dinsmore WW. Detection of human papilloma virus DNA sequences in oral squamous cell papillomas by the polymerase chain reaction. Oral Surg Oral Med Oral Pathol Oral Radiol Endod 1995;80(1):63-6.

Williams JD, Sclafani AP, Slupchinskij O, Douge C. Evaluation and management of the lingual thyroid gland. Ann Otol Rhinol Laryngol 1996;105(4):312-6.

Williams WJ, Beutler E, Eislev AJ, et al. Hematology, 4th edn. New York: McGraw-Hill, 1990. Wilkin's dental practice of dental hygienist. Williams and Wilkin's: Lippincot. 8th edn. 1999.pp.342-5.

Wood NK, Goaz PW. Differential diagnosis of oral and maxillofacial lesions. Mosby company. 5th edn. 1997.

Wright BA, Fenwick F. Candidiasis and atrophic tongue lesions. Oral Surg Oral Med Oral Pathol 1981;51(1):55-61.

Wu WC, Schifftner TL, Henderson WG, et al. Preoperative hematocrit levels and postoperative outcomes in older patients undergoing noncardiac surgery. J Am Med Assoc 2007;297(22):2481-8.

Zakrzewska JM, Forssell H, Glenny AM. Interventions for the treatment of burning mouth syndrome. Cochrane Database Syst Rev 2005;(1):CD002779.

Zarb GA, Bergman B, Payton JA, et al. Prosthodontic treatment for partially edentulous patients. St. Louis: CV Mosby Co, 1978.

Zargari O. The prevalence and significance of fissured tongue and geographical tongue in psoriatic patients. Clin Exp Dermatol 2006;31(2):192-5.

Index

Page numbers followed by *t* refer to table.

A

Aarskog syndrome 34
Abscess 203
Abutment 203
Accessory nerve 21
Acetaminophen 132
Acetylsalicylic acid 164
Acid etching 203
Acquired immune deficiency syndrome 160
Actinomycosis 128
Acupuncture 139
Acyclovir 121, 137
Addison's disease 36
Adenoid facies 39
Adipose tissue 28
Adrenal insufficiency 157, 163
Air borne fungi 105
Alanine transaminase 154
Alban test 98
Albright's disease 36, 54
Alcohol consumption 25
Alcoholism 24
Alfalfa 141
Allergy 22, 163, 168
Alveoloplasty 204
Amalgam 204
- restorations, large 59

Ammonia 193
Amoebiasis 11
Amoxicillin 121
Amphotericin 122
Ampicillin 122
Analgesia 204
Anaphylaxis 168
Ancillary 204
Anemia 36, 48, 67, 150
- hemolytic 150
- signs of 32

Anesthetic testing 73
Angina 15, 170
Angioedema 129
Angle's class
- I malocclusion 61
- II malocclusion 61

Ankyloglossia 49
Anodontia 56
Antibiotic 164
- prophylaxis regimens 149*t*
- sensitivity test 77

Antifibrinolytic agents 128
Antiglobulin test 109
Antihistamine 129
Anxiety reduction 167
Anxiolysis 204
Apexification 204
Apexogenesis 204
Aphthosis, simple 135
Aphthous ulcer 46
Apical abscess, acute 203
Apicoectomy 204
Arch 204
Areata migrans 49
Aromatherapy 143
Artifacts, types of 104
Ascher's syndrome 46
Aspiration 167
Aspirin 164
- burn, causes of 120

Asthma 15, 169
- attacks 167
- management 169
- signs of acute severe 169

Auer bodies 82
Augmentin 122
Auspitz sign 36
Autogenous graft 204

B

Bacterial
- diseases 11
- endocarditis, subacute 16

Basophilic stippling 82
Behçet's disease 129

Behçet's syndrome 34
Benzocaine 125
Benzodiazepines 23, 153
Benzyl penicillin 123
Betamethasone phosphate tablets 127
Biological therapy 143
Biopsy 98
  punches 102
Bite
  closed 206
  deep 206
  open 219
  test 73
Bitewing
  radiograph 113, 205
  vertical 230
Bitot's spots 34
Black
  hairy tongue 49
  hyperpigmentation, causes of 186
Bleaching 205
Bleeding 12
  disorders 151
  time, determination of 85
Blood
  agar media 93
  dyscrasias 51
  glucose, postprandial 89
  pressure 29, 30, 158, 200
    diastolic 200
    systolic 200
  sugar
  estimation of 88
    high 15
    low 15
  transfusions 22
Body
  build physique 28
  fluid, chemistry of 196
  mass index 200, 201
  temperature 32, 201
Bone marrow aspiration 87
Boxer's nose 34
Breath, shortness of 16
Breathing 166
  difficulty during 163
  problems 15
Bronchial asthma 152
Bronchiectasis 35
Brown sclera 34
Brush biopsy 103
  artifact 104
  procedure 104
Bruxism 205
Buccal mucosa 50, 51*t*
Bupivacaine 125, 157
Burning sensation 12, 185
Burns 36
Burr cells 82

C

Cabot ring 82
Canal, mandibular 217
Cancer 15, 24, 67
  bowel 24
  breast 24
  ovarian 24
Candida albicans 106
Candida infections 129
Canines, mandibular 194
Cantilever extension 205
Capillary fragility test 87
Carbon dioxide snow 71
Cardiac ailments 163
Cardiac arrest 171
  management 171
  signs 171
Cardiac contraction 29
Cardiac disorders 6
Cardiac markers 200
Cardiac problems 147
Cardiopulmonary resuscitation 165
Cardiovascular disease 120
Caries 206
  activity tests 95
  classification of 60
  detecting dyes 69
Carious lesion 206
Carmellose gelatin paste 127
Castleman's disease 43
Cat-scratch disease 190
Cavity 206
  test 73
Cell volume
  determination of packed 79
  mean 81
Cellulitis 206
Cementoenamel junction 54
Cementum 206
Central nervous system disorders 25
Cephadroxil 124
Cephalexin 124
Cephalosporins 124, 164
Cerebral spinal fluid 200
Chamomile 141

Cheek 189
Cheilitis glandularis 130
Cheilitis granulomatosa 130
Chemotherapy 163
Chest pain 17
Chickenpox 15
Childhood illnesses, chronic 15
Chloasma gravidarum 36
Choking 167
Cholera 11
Cholesterol 15, 193
Chromosome analysis 111
Cigarette smoker's lip 46
Circulatory system 29
Clark's rule 10
Cleft
  palate 206
  tongue 49
Clenching 206
Clindamycin 124, 129
Clot retraction time, determination of 85
Clotrimazole 130
Clotting time, determination of 85
Cloves 141
Cold
  abscess 45
  air, spray with 70
  test 70
  water bath 71
Colorimetric Snyder test 96
Complex aphthosis 136
Compound fracture 207
Congestive cardiac failure 16
Coombs test 109
Coronary heart disease 35
Corpuscular hemoglobin, mean 81
Corticosteroid sparing systemic therapy 134
Cosmetic dentistry 208
Cough 17
Coumadine 164
Coumarin derivatives 22
Cranial nerve examination 20
Creamy-yellow plaques 33
Creatinine 193
Crohn's disease 35
Crossbite 208
Crown 208
  artificial 204
  clinical 206
  lengthening 208
Cushing's disease 36
Cushing's syndrome 29, 34, 39
Cusp 208
Cyanosis, signs of 33
Cyst 208
Cytomegalovirus 190

D

Dapsone 133
Darier's disease 35
Deciduous dentition 210
Dementia 195
Dental 204
  caries 12, 60
  fluorosis 58
  history, past 14
  medicine 4
  office 146
  physical therapy treatment 144*t*
  practitioners 2
  procedure 149*t*, 156
  terminology, current 208
  treatment 155, 163*t*, 164*t*
Dentin dysplasia 58
Dentistry
  drugs in 120
  evidence-based 212
  preventive 224
Dentition
  adult 203, 223
  mixed 218
  transitional 229
Dentofacial orthopedics 221
Denture 210
  base 210
  fixed partial 213
  immediate 215
  partial 222
  removable partial 225
  stomatitis 51
  temporary removable 228
  wearers 51
Deoxyhemoglobin 33
Depression 24
Dexamethasone sodium phosphate 127
Diabetes 15, 36, 62, 163
  mellitus 24, 67, 147, 159
    symptoms of 147
Diastema 210
Diazepam 23, 125, 174
Dietary habit 26
Dietary supplements 138
Diffusion test 77
Digitalis 164

Digoxine 164
Dilantin 164
Dilling rule 10
Dilution test 78
Dip slide method 97
Discectomy 210
Disease
 control, center for 155
 expressed in families 24*t*
 malignant 43
Dohle bodies 82
Down's syndrome 29, 34, 39, 49
Doxepin 129
Doxycycline 123, 129
Dry mouth 12
 causes of 185
 drugs with 185
Dry socket 211

E

Eating nails, habit of 35
Ecchymosis 211
Ectopic eruption 211
Electrical stimulation 144
Enamel 211
 hypoplasia 58
 solubility test 97
Endocarditis prophylaxis 148, 149
Endocrine
 diseases 43
 system 18
Energy therapy 145
Enzyme-linked immunosorbent assay (ELISA) 110
Eosinophil count, absolute 84
Epilepsy 15, 152, 163, 171
 management 172
 signs 172
 symptoms 172
Epinephrine 121
Epstein-Barr virus 45
Eruption sequestrum 58
Erythema 19, 211
 multiforme 131
Erythematous lesions 211
Erythrocyte
 indices, determination of 80
 sedimentation rate 80, 196
Escherichia coli 11
Ethyl chloride 71
Eucalyptus 141
Exfoliative cytology 101
 advantages 102
 disadvantages 102
 procedure 101
Extremities 35
Eye 33, 136
 blinking of 34

F

Facebow 212
Facial 212
 droop 16
 nerve 21
 pain, atypical 13
 profile 38
Fascia 212
Fasting blood sugar 89
Fever 36
Fiberotomy 213
Fine needle aspiration biopsy 99
 advantages 100
 procedure 100
Finger nails, clubbing of 35
Fistulous track 213
Fluconazole 125
Flumazenil 174
Focal epithelial hyperplasia 46
Folic acid deficiency 48
Frenectomy 213
Frenum 213
Frey's hair 21
Frozen sections 105
 advantages 105
 procedure 105

G

Gait 28
Gastric ulcers 120
Gastrointestinal diseases 25
Gastrointestinal system 17
Genetic test 213
Giant cell arteritis 13
Gingiva 53, 189, 214
 free 53
Gingival crevice, microbial flora from 95
Gingival pemphigoid 134
Gingival sulcus 53
 depth of 55
Gingivectomy 214
Gingivitis 214

Gingivoplasty 214
Gland specific saliva 107
Glass ionomer 214
Glaucoma 163
Glucocorticoid therapy 156
  type of 156
Glucose 193
  tolerance test 90
Glycosylated hemoglobin 91
Gold foil 214
Gummy smile 214

H

Haemophilus influenzae 109
Hairy tongue 48, 132
Halitosis 12
  causes of 186
Hard palate 189
Hard tissue
  examination 55
  imaging 116
Hashimoto's thyroiditis 18
Head and neck region, examination of 38
Hearing loss 195
Heart 30
  attacks 15
  failure, right sided 42
  rate 200
Heat test 71
Hematocrit 79
Hematologic values, normal 196
Hemoglobin 79, 196
  electrophoresis 87
  determination of 79
Hemophilia 6, 24, 151, 163
Hemorrhagic tendencies 6
Hemostasis, disorders of 120
Hemotocrit 196
Hepatic disorders 36
Hepatitis
  A 11
  B 11, 154, 190
  C 11
Herbst appliance 214
Herpangina 132
Herpes labialis 46
Herpes zoster 132
Herpetic gingivostomatitis, acute 128
Heterophile test 109
Hoarseness 17
Hormonal imbalance 36
Howell-Jolly bodies 82
Human immunodeficiency virus 160
  infection 190
Hydrocortisone
  acetate 127
  hemisuccinate pellets 126
Hydroxychloroquine 133
Hypercholesterolemia 15
Hyperdontia 56
Hyperlipidemia 24, 33
Hypertension 14, 24, 163
Hyperthyroidism 39
Hyperventilation 163, 167
Hypnosis 140
Hypochromic cells 82
Hypoglossal nerve 21
Hypoglycemia 171, 173
  management 173
  signs 173
  symptoms 173
Hypopituitarism 36
Hypotension 163
Hypothyroidism 39
Hypoxia 171

I

Ibuprofen 121, 132
Ice therapy 144
Incisal angle 215
Incisors, mandibular 194
Inflammation, acute 41
Inhibits warfarin metabolism 151
Initial emergency procedures 165
Insulin 164
Intentional reimplantation 215
Interim prosthesis 215
International classification of diseases 215
Intra-articular corticosteroids 127
Intracranial hypertension, benign 13
Intralesional corticosteroids 127
Intralesional therapy 133
Intraoral imaging 112
Iodine preparations 69
Iron
  binding capacity 87
  deficiency 48
Ischemic heart disease 14, 24
Itraconazole 125

J

Jaundice 17, 163
Jaw 216
  jerk 21
  lower 217
  medical management of 4
Jegher's syndrome 54

K

Kawasaki disease 43, 45, 190
Keratin 216
Keratinized gingiva 216
Keratotic lesion 216
Ketoacidosis 48
Ketoconazole 126, 157
Keyes biopsy punch 102
Kikuchi's disease 43
Klinefelter's syndrome 29
Koebner's phenomenon 36
Kyphosis 29

L

Labial mucosa 50, 51*t*
Laminate veneer 216
Lanoxine 164
Laser Doppler flowmetry 74
Leong's premolar 57
Leonine facies 39
Leprosy 34
Lesion 216
  red 51
  white 51
Leukemia 18, 190
Leukocyte count, differential 83, 197
Leukonychia 35
Lichen planus 132
Lidocaine, topical 132
Life-threatening asthma, signs of 169
Lignocaine 126
Lindblom's view 116
Linea alba buccalis 50
Lingua nigra 49
Lingual thyroid 49
Lip 46, 189
  bumper 216
  incompetence 217
Lipid storage disease 43
Liver
  disorders 153
  function test 154
Local anesthesia 217
Lontophoresis 144
Lordosis 29
Lotrimin 130
Ludwig's angina 45
Lugol's iodine staining 75
Lung
  abscess 35
  disease 6
Lupus erythematosus 133, 190
Lyme disease 11
Lymph nodes, consistencies of 44*t*
Lymphadenitis
  acute 44
  chronic 44
Lymphadenopathy
  causes of 42, 43*t*, 190
  evaluation of 190
Lymphoma 18
Lymphosarcoma 44
Lysozyme 193

M

Macrodontia 56
Macroglossia 49
Macrolides 164
Macule 217
Malaria 11, 150
Malignant neoplasm, TNM classification of 192
Malocclusion 217
Mandibular
  anterior 195
  cross-sectional 195
  lateral 195
  occlusal projections 194
Marfan's syndrome 29, 34
Maryland bridge 217
Massage therapy 144
Masses 217
Masseter muscle 41
Mastication, muscle of 41
Maxilla 217
Maxillary
  anterior 194
  canines 194
  cross-sectional 194
  incisors 194
  lateral 194
  molars 194
  occlusal projections 194
  premolars 194

Measles 15
Medical emergencies 161
  drugs for 195
  management of 161
Melkersson-Rosenthal syndrome 47
Membrane, barrier 204
Meningitis 11
Methylprednisolone acetate 127
Metronidazole 123
Microabrasion 218
Microdontia 56
Microglossia 49
Midazolam 174
Migraine 24
Migratory glossitis, benign 49
Mikulicz's syndrome 39
Mind-body interventions 139
Moist heat 144
Molar 218
  mandibular 194
Mononucleosis-type syndromes 190
Mouth, floor of 52, 189
Mouthguard 218
Mucogingival junction 53
Mucous membrane 51, 219
Mumps 15
Muscle 40
  spasm 40
Muscular dystrophy 39
Musculoskeletal pain 121
Musculoskeletal system 19
Mycobacterium antibodies 110
Mycobacterium tuberculosis 160
Myocardial infarction 170
Myofascial pain disorder syndrome 42
Myopia 24
Myxedema 35, 36

N

Nail 35
Neck, examination of 42
Necrotizing ulcerative gingivitis, acute 55, 128
Nerve
  auditory 21
  blocking, diagnostic 77
Neural transmission, interference with 77
Neurologic diseases 24
Neurologic system 19
Neurological disorders 13
Neutralization test 109
Nevus 133
Niacin 48
  deficiency 48
Niacinamide 134
Nikolsky's sign 36
Nitrobide 164
Nitroglycerin 164
Nitrostate 164
Noonan's syndrome 29
Nose 34
Nuclear medicine 118
Numbness 12
Nutrition 143
Nutritional deficiency 48
Nystatin 126
  oral suspension 130

O

Obstructive pulmonary disease, chronic 46
Occlusal radiographs 113
Odontogenic
  cyst 219
  pain 12
  tumors 190
Odontoplasty 219
Office emergency plan 162
Olfactory nerve 20
Onychophagia 35
Optic nerve 20
Ora test 98
Oral and maxillofacial
  pathologist 220
  pathology 220
  radiologist 220
  radiology 220
  surgeon 220
  surgery 220
Oral brown hyperpigmentation, causes of 186
Oral cavity 190
  habits to 25
  lymphatic drainage of 189
Oral diseases 12
  treatment of common 128
Oral health literacy 220
Oral lesions, management of 134
Oral malignant neoplasms 191
Oral medicine 1, 3, 4
Oral microbial flora 93
Oral mucosa, medical management of 4
Oral ulcers, causes of 188
Organ transplants 163

Orofacial pain, causes of 13*t*
Oropharynx 52
Orthodontic 221
  appliance, removable 225
  device 221
  retainer 221
Orthopnea 16
Osteomyelitis, cases of 65
Osteoplasty 221
Osteoporosis 24
Osteotomy 221
Ovarian failure 18

P

Packed cell volume 196
Pain 12
  management of 121
Palatal expander 221
Palate 51, 221
Palmar erythema 35
Palsy 19
Pancreatitis 25
Papilla 221
Paralysis 19
Paranormal health remedies 140
Paraparesis 19
Parasite disease 11
Paresthesia 12, 19
Parkinson's disease 39
Parotid papillae 51
Passavant's bar 52
Pediatric
  dentist 222
  dentistry 222
Pemphigoid 134
Pemphigus vulgaris 134
Penciclovir cream 136
Penicillin 22, 164
  G 122
  V 122
Peptic ulcer 25
  contraindicated in 121
Periapical abscess, chronic 206
Periapical cyst 222
Periodontal disease 222
Periodontal pocket 223
Periodontium 223
Peripheral blood smear, examination of 81
Peripheral edema 16
Periradicular abscess 203
Permanent dentition 223
Pernicious anemia 150
Peutz-Jegher syndrome 36
Phenytoin 164
Phonophoresis 144
Plaque
  disclosing agents 69
  microbial flora from 95
Plaquenil 133
Plasma
  cell gingivitis 135
  count, determination of 85
Plummer-Vinson syndrome 35
Polio 11, 15
Postherpetic neuralgia 132
Prednisolone sodium phosphate 127
Prednisone 133
Pregnancy 23, 36, 163
Premature eruption 58
Premolars, mandibular 194
Prosthesis 224
  fixed-removable 213
Prosthetic joint
  infections, prevention of 160*t*
  replacement 158
Prosthodontic 224
  retainer 224
Prosthodontist 224
Protein 193
Prothrombin time, determination of 86
Protozoan disease 11
Psychiatric disease 19
Pterygoid
  lateral 41
  medial 41
Public health dentistry 224
Pulmonary disease 163
Pulp 224
  Cap
    direct 210
    indirect 215
  cavity 225
  oximetry 74
  tests, electric 72
  vitality tests 70
Pulpectomy 225
Pulpitis 225
Pulpotomy 225
Pulse 30, 200
Punch biopsy 102
  advantages 103
  disadvantages 103
  technique 103
Punctal occlusion 136
Pupils, asymmetrical 20

R

Rabies 11
Radiation
  induced mucositis 135
  therapy 163
Radiolucency-radiopacity, mixed 218
Red blood cell count 82, 197
Red lesions, causes of 187
Regional odontodysplasia 58
Renal
  diseases 153
  failure 36, 153
Residual root 226
Resorption
  external 59
  internal 59
Respiratory rate 31, 201
Respiratory system 17
Restoration
  direct 210
  indirect 215
Reticulocyte count 197
  determination of 84
Rheumatic fever 15
Rhomboid glossitis, median 49
Riboflavin deficiency 48
Rinne's test 21
Root 226
  canal 226
    therapy 226
Ropivacaine 126
Rubella 15
Rubinstein-Taybi syndrome 57

S

Sacral edema 16
Saliva
  mixed 107
  substitute 126
  whole 107
Salivary
  buffer capacity test 97
  flow test 76
  gland 226
    damage to 77
    diseases 118
    medical management of 4
    swelling, causes of 191
  reductase test 97
  Streptococcus mutans level test 97
  swelling 62
Salmonella 11
Salmonella typhi
  H 109
  O 109
Sarcoidosis 190
Scarlet fever 15, 48
Schilling's test 87
Schistosomiasis 11
Sclera 33
Scleroderma dystrophy 39
Scoliosis 29
Seizures 167
Sensation, abnormal 19
Sensitivity test 208
Serum fibrinogen 88
Serum iron 87
Shepherd's purse 142
Shigella 11
Sialoadenitis 119
Sialochemical investigations 106
Sialodochoplasty 227
Sialography 118
Sialolithotomy 227
Sialosis 62
Sickle cell preparation 87
Sinus problems 163
Sjögren's syndrome 34, 39, 119, 136
Smell, perversion of 20
Smoker's palate 51
Smoker's patch 51
Soft palate 189
Sores 12
Specimen collection procedure 93
Spur cells 82
Sputum 17
Squamous cell carcinoma 46
Steroid cover, estimation of 157*t*
Steroid therapy 155
Steven-Johnson syndrome 34, 137
Still man's clefts 228
Stomatitis 228
Streptococcal pharyngitis 190
Streptococcus mutans 97, 106
  screening test 98
Streptococcus pyogenes 109
Sublingual dermoid cyst 45
Sulfa drugs 22
Sulfonamides 22, 164
Swab test 96
Swelling 12, 181, 191
  examination of 62
Syncope 167, 172
  management 173

signs 173
symptoms 173
Syphilis 67
Syphilitic hypoplasia 58
Syphilitic ulcers 50
Systemic corticosteroids 130
Systemic diseases 67
Systemic lupus erythemateus 108
Systolic blood pressure 147

T

Talon's cusp 57
Taurodontism 57
Tea tree oil 142
Teeth 62, 189, 225
apices, cultures of 94
bounded space 228
discoloration of 59
displaced 210
eruption, delayed 12
impacted 215
loose 12
multiple unerupted 58
supernumerary 228
syndrome, cracked 208
transplantation of 229
wear 59
Temazepam 23
Temporalis 41
Temporomandibular disorders 27
Temporomandibular joint 39, 77, 228
dysfunction 228
examination 39
radiography 115
disorders of 42
Tetanus 11
Tetracycline 23, 123, 134
Thalassemia 39
Thalidomide 23
Thermal pulp tests 70
Thiamine 48
Thrombin time, determination of 86
Thromboplastin time, partial 86
Thyme 142
Thyroglossal cyst 45
Thyroid isthmus, goiter of 45
Tissue
conditioning 228
regeneration 214
Tobacco
consumption 24
excessive use of 59
Toludine blue 75
Tongue 47, 189
anomalies of 49
crib 228
fissured 49, 131
geographic 48, 49, 131
scrotal 49
thrust 228
tie 49
ulcerations of 50
Tonsils 189
Total leukocyte count 83, 197
Tourniquet test 87
Toxoplasmosis 190
Tracheotomy 229
Traditional Chinese medicine 138
Tranexamic acid 128
Transcranial projection 116
Transcutaneous electrical nerve stimulator 144
Transorbital projection 116
Traumatic ulcer 46
Triamcinolone
acetonide 127
hexacetonide 127
Trigeminal nerve 20
Trypanosomiasis 11
Tuberculosis 15, 67, 137, 160, 163
lymphadenitis 44, 190
Tuberosity 229
Tumor 40
benign 119
Turner's hypoplasia 58
Turner's syndrome 29

U

Ulcer 182
acute 50
chronic 50
examination of 63
Ulcerative colitis 35
Ulcerative lesions 46
Urea 193
Uremia, advanced 48
Uric acid 193
Urine
analysis 199
blood sugar 92
values, normal 199

V

Vagus nerve 21
van der Woude syndrome 47

Vancomycin 124
Varicosities 230
Vascular disorders 13
Vasocoolant spray 144
Vesiculobullous disorders 188
Viral diseases 11
Vital signs 29, 162, 200
Vitamin
  A deficiency 48
  B_{12} 150
    deficiency 150
Vomiting preventive 141
von Recklinghausen disease 54

W

Waardenburg syndrome 34
Waldeyer's ring 52
Warfarin 164
Weber's test 21
Wegener's granulomatosis 137
Wheeze 17
Whooping cough 15
Widal test 109
Wintrobe's constants 80

X

Xerostomia 77, 230

Y

Yeast 230
Yellow fever 11
Young's rule 10

Z

Zimmer's projection 116
Zosteriform 36
Zygomatic bone 230